Friendly Microbiome

Food and Beverages Which Are Beneficial to a Healthy Gut, and Ways to Implement Them Into Your Diet and Everyday Life

JOHN SALUTELLI

*For all the people who,
while pursuing a specific goal,
found something else...*

TABLE OF CONTENTS

Introduction _____ 9

What Are Microbiomes? _____ 10

Why Is the Microbiome Important? _____ 11

Let's Get Going _____ 12

Chapter 1: Healthy Gut Microbiome _____ 14

Dietary Fiber _____ 15

Immune System _____ 16

Mental Health _____ 18

Research and Science _____ 19

In Summary _____ 20

Chapter 2: Unhealthy Gut Microbiome _____ 22

Stomach Issues _____ 23

Sugar _____ 26

Sleeping Issues _____ 30

In Summary _____ 31

Chapter 3: Improving Your Gut Microbiome _____ 32

Restoring Gut Flora _____ 34

Naturally Increasing Good Bacteria _____ 35

Exercise _____ 37

Intermittent Fasting _____ 38

Alcohol _____ 39

Quick Fix Diets _____ 40

In Summary _____ 41

Chapter 4: The Importance of a Healthy Lifestyle _____ 42

Benefits of a Healthy Lifestyle _____ 43

One Step at a Time _____ 48

Personal Care _____ 50

In Summary _____ 51

Chapter 5: Rebooting Your Microbiome _____ 52

Boosting Your Microbiome _____ 54

Improving Digestion _____ 58

In Summary _____ 62

Chapter 6: Microbiome Enriched Foods _____ 63

Probiotics and Prebiotics _____ 65

Chapter 7: Microbiome-Friendly Food Groups _____ 70

Vegetables _____ 71

Grains _____ 73

Fruit _____ 76

Dairy _____ 79

Fats _____ 80

Protein _____ 82

Herbs and Spices _____ 84

Chapter 8: Lifestyle Options And Sample Meal Plans _____ 87

Mediterranean Diet _____ 89

The Paleo Diet _____ 95

Low-Carb Diet _____ 100

The Vegan Lifestyle _____ 104

The Microbiome Diet _____ 110

In Summary _____ 116

Chapter 9: Recipes _____ 118

Breakfast _____ 119

Lunch _____ 121

Dinner _____ 124

Dessert/Snacks _____ 128

Fermentation Guide _____ 132

Conclusion _____ 134

Our Promise _____ 135

Food for Thought _____ 136

Be Kind to Yourself _____ 136

It Is Time... _____ 137

About The Author _____ 138

References _____ 140

Introduction

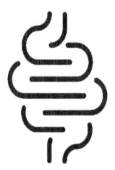

Oh great, yet another book trying to force you into following another diet. Just another dust collector on the bookshelf, or a space filler on your kindle. There are thousands of different diets floating around which are backed by science, doctors, dieticians, clinicians, and even celebrities. There are diet clubs and groups all around the world which intimidate you into losing a certain amount of ounces and pounds while being weighed in front of your fellow dieters. Most, if not all of us, have been around this block a number of times, had the t-shirts, and burned them. Dieting might come naturally to some people, eating the right amount of this, that and the other, and the pounds just melt away. We try diets and follow them to the letter but we end up gaining weight instead of losing, which is most disheartening. What worked for Jane might not work for Sarah because no two people are the same.

The aim of this book is to help you gain insight into what is going on in your body. Yes, we all know that our bodies are home to all our vital organs, where everything fits together like a puzzle. We know that the blood flows through our veins to help keep these organs ticking and churning. We are well aware that the average body consists of up to 60% water thanks to the health lessons at school. We also know that we have to look after our bodies by taking care of what we consume, whether it be food, drinks, or medication.

With this book, we want to help you understand, and possibly even help you to make positive changes. There will be a selection of diets, meal plans, and recipes to suit various types of lifestyles. No one can force you to do anything you do not want to do. We are going to present you with all the information we have gathered while putting this book together. There will be a smattering of scientific explanations, but do not fear, these will be used to loop us all into what is happening inside our bodies. They will help you understand why normal diets don't typically work for different individuals. At the end of the day, you will be able to weigh up the pros and cons and make an informed decision for you and your health. There will be no sugarcoating and no quick fixes, as this is a lifestyle change. There will be no bullying because we all know that bullying breaks down your self-confidence, and we do not want that.

What Are Microbiomes?

What in the world are microbiomes? This is where we will call in the help of scientists. When we are born, our tiny bodies are exposed to trillions of microbes. These microbes make their home in and on our bodies. According to scientists, the microbes are a community of healthy bacteria, viruses, microscopic bugs, and fungi. These critters, in their collective, are referred to as the microbiome.

We all have our very own, personally tailored conglomerate of microbes that are unique to us. No two people have the same collection of microbes. This makes our microbiome's DNA unique and sets us apart from everyone else.

Wait! What? There are critters inside my body? Your first thought is probably trying to figure out how to get rid of them quickly and painlessly. Settle down. Take a deep breath and continue reading. These critters are necessary for your health and well-being. If you are alive and breathing today, then you should know that these critters are doing a bang-up job keeping everything working. The microbiome performs a pretty nifty function in our bodies. After years of ongoing research, it has been determined that the bacteria in us are beneficial to our bodies and lives. These microbes aid us in various ways, such as digesting food, building up and strengthening our immune systems, and producing the necessary vitamins to help our bodies cope. In short, they protect us from any harmful bacterial entities that try to invade our bodies. While you might be doing everything in your power to stay healthy, there are harmful bacteria that will and do slip through the cracks.

Why Is the Microbiome Important?

As previously mentioned, our bodies play host to a community of microbes that are tailor-made for us. The microbiomes live on and in various parts of our bodies such as the skin, the mouth, and the intestines. Over the course of time, these microbiomes will grow, mature, and change to accommodate any changes to our lifestyles and diets. As time moves on, you will adopt new microbes. This is part of keeping up with the trends called life. You will be introduced to new foods, and you will interact with people from all walks of life, which will help your microbiome grow and become accustomed to any and all changes.

In other words, your microbiomes will become more specialized and equipped to ward off harmful bacteria and viruses. It is fascinating to realize that your microbiome will not stop growing and changing until you reach a ripe old age. While this might seem like devastating news, it does not mean it is bad news for us. Remember, science has proven that your microbiome is a part of you and your existence. As we age, as with everything in life, things slow down. When you are born, you do not come with an expiration date. Make the most of your life, and live life to the fullest.

Let's Get Going

You thought you were going to get a science lesson on microbes and microbiomes. This might be a little bit true, but this is not that kind of book. We wanted to give you the basics so that you can understand how things work without scientific calculations and diagrams that will leave you with more questions than answers. There are more than enough books that give you scientific names and explanations that will blow your mind. The aim here is to help you understand the basics of what goes on in our bodies.

As already mentioned, no one is going to force you into doing anything you do not want to do. We really would appreciate it if you will join us until the end. We will not give you a list of medications that you will need. As with any dietary changes, consult with your medical practitioner or specialist. This book will take on a holistic approach. We will present you with various foods, beverages, exercises, and tips and tricks which can help your microbiome grow and be healthy. Simple changes to your lifestyle could impact your health greatly.

While changing your lifestyle will improve your microbiome, dropping a few pounds along the way will be a huge bonus. Health is the number one takeaway from changing the way we adapt to a new lifestyle. You will notice that you will be spending less at the local drugstore because you are feeling energized and revitalized. Your energy levels will increase. This is all exciting, especially if you have been struggling with your health for quite some time.

Chapter 1: Healthy Gut Microbiome

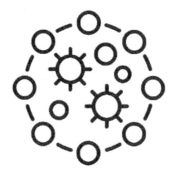

With the help of scientists, we have determined that our bodies contain communities of microbes that live on our skin, in our mouths, and in our guts. The foods we eat from birth, whether breastfed or formula-fed, play a role in how our gut microbiome works. As we get older and introduce a variety of different foods, our microbiome is consistently adapting to keep up with the changes. This is normal in order to build up our systems to cope with all the different types of food we eat, condiments we use, and beverages we consume.

The microbes in our intestines and stomach are very important to our overall well-being and health. Have you ever thought about what goes on in your body when you eat or drink something? What goes on in the inside of our bodies can be likened to a processing factory.

There are different departments within our stomach and intestines. The foods we eat, and there are many different types, all go through a department where they are broken down. Our little critters work overtime to make sure everything works like a well-oiled machine.

We are going to take a look at some of the functions of the departments of our internal factory. Before we can move on to the do's and don'ts of what we consume, we should start with the basics. The basics are understanding what goes on under the hood. Once you understand how everything works, you will be better equipped to implement any changes.

Dietary Fiber

Your microbiome aids in digesting fiber which is essential to your gut by producing the important short-chain fatty acids. There are numerous health benefits when eating fiber which play an important role in your overall well-being, such as reducing the chance of cardiovascular disease and lowering body weight. We are not telling you to go out and buy all kinds of fiber-related foodstuffs and supplements. Fiber comes from fruit, vegetables, and other sources. Healthy fiber, when eaten in the right amounts, can prevent you from gaining weight and regulate your blood sugar.

Fiber is a form of carbohydrates which is beneficial to our bodies. Thinking in terms of various types of diets, many deter you from eating carbohydrates. Not many understand this concept because on the one hand, scientists and dieticians are telling us to eat carbohydrates, but on the other, they're telling us not to eat them. Unless explained to you in simple layman's terms, you will be confused forever and decide to give up before even thinking of changing how you eat. We will be discussing various types of diets later in this book, but for now, we are trying to understand the meanings and terminology of what is going on inside our bodies.

As already mentioned, fiber is found in fresh fruit and vegetables. These are unprocessed carbohydrates. This means that they have not gone through the process of being modified to be preserved, cooked, have additives added, and so forth before you get to consume them. These unprocessed carbohydrates are literally from the ground, tree, or plant to our tables where we can add our own condiments, fats, or however else we enjoy our produce. Processed carbohydrates are those that have been broken down. This comes in the form of flour, pasta, rice, corn, and many more. Although the ingredients are listed on the packaging, we will not know for sure how much fiber or good nutrients are in the products.

No one is going to tell you what to eat and what not to eat because you have a will and mind of your own. You are not a robot that will or can be dictated to. You are merely being given different options to help you decide what is best suited to your current needs and lifestyle. Do not feel too guilty about eating those five slices of deliciously home-baked sourdough bread just yet. We are only at the beginning stages of figuring out how your gut microbiome would like you to treat it. The best is yet to come.

Immune System

If you look at yourself in the mirror, you will see your reflection. You blink your eyes, you twitch your nose, or you make funny faces, and your reflection mimics your actions. Unfortunately for us, we can't see what is going on inside our bodies. We know things are happening inside us because science has told us this. We have a feeling of something brewing and churning inside our bodies. Well, as already mentioned many times since we started on this epic journey, our bodies are home to a community of bacteria, fungi, and viruses. We have learned that this community helps keep us healthy by constantly growing to keep up with our daily needs.

It is fascinating to learn how everything works in layman's terms since many of us do not get the concept of science and we are no medical professionals. At the most, we tend to pretend we are WebMD or Google doctors where we search for symptoms and possible cures. More than that, and we are as clueless as a snail running a marathon.

As mentioned in the previous section, our bodies are basically processing factories. When you eat or drink something, it goes through a selection process to determine what belongs where. From there, it is sent on to other departments to either add to the community or turn them into something useful such as antibodies. After the processes have been completed, the waste is expelled from our bodies through secretion. Unfortunately, some harmful bacteria, viruses, or fungi slip through the cracks, and we end up sick.

This is where our established and ever-growing microbiome gets to work. Our personalized army of microbes stands together to block these invaders. This personalized army is part of our immune system. It is important to realize that in order to have a healthy immune system, one that will fight off and protect us from these harmful invaders, we need to take in a healthy diet. It might sound easier said than done, but everyone is different in how they ward off infections and diseases. A healthy immune system can easily be broken, through no fault of our own, but by following a healthy lifestyle, we are able to contain and/or minimize these attacks.

Even though we might be following a healthy lifestyle and doing all we can to keep ourselves protected, there is no guarantee that you will not get sick. All it takes is one bite or a sip of something, no matter how healthy or unhealthy that may be, for the army inside your body to start fighting for you. Unhealthy bacteria can thrive on healthy bodies and will stop at nothing to make your life miserable. It is not a reflection on you or your lifestyle should that happen. This is all part of the circle of life.

Mental Health

Who would have thought that what we put into our mouths would make its way to our brain? By now we know that the community of critters living inside us wants what is best for us. They break down the things we consume and send them along their way to all the right places so that they can fulfill their tasks at keeping us healthy from the inside. The breaking down of food in our intestines produces metabolites that have an influence on all the cells in our bodies, including the nervous system.

This is where our healthy immune systems come into play. Whatever harmful bacteria might filter through our system undetected will produce molecules. These molecules can affect how our brains deal with situations. In order for normal cognitive and emotional processing to occur, a healthy microbiome is very important to ensure we are happy. What happens is that your microbiome interacts with your central nervous system, the brain, and the spinal cord. This is known as endocrine and immune signaling triggers.

Scientists have been researching the relationship between the gut microbiome and brain since the early 1970s. While research is still ongoing, and will probably continue until the end of ages, there is no clear knowledge of how the gut microbiome and the central nervous system actually work together. There has, however, been proof that changes in the gut can result in an increased intestinal activity and that neuroactive compounds do enter the blood. Research has also proven that the changes in our microbiota can cause depression, affect how we cope with different social interactions, and protect the immune system from stressful situations.

Your dynamic microbiome sets you apart from the next person. Whatever triggers your friends' moods might not be the same for you. As you already know, your microbiome is unique to you, this cannot be stressed enough, and you cannot compare your symptoms or lack thereof to anyone else.

If eating chocolate makes you happy, it might have the opposite effect on someone else. This could be due to the fact that they have an aversion to something in that chocolate because their microbiome setup is different. This is a trial and error of what food, beverages, or medication your body can tolerate. Your gut will alert you the moment it is not happy. Listen to your gut, and it can tell you a lot.

Research and Science

The human microbiome is a subject that has been studied over many years to try and understand what role your gut plays in your health. There are over a trillion microbes in each microbiome and it is impossible for scientists to research each and every one because the bacteria, viruses, and fungi are ever-changing. This will not deter them from trying to figure out all that is going on inside us. The research will continue for years to come and will give scientists endless opportunities to understand how these critters work and possibly prevent illnesses that could claim our lives.

It is impossible to offer a timeline for the research due to the dynamics of day-to-day living. What was thought to be a cure two years ago could have changed because of the way food is being processed today. Yes, whatever you consume plays a major factor in what goes on in your body. Even interacting with friends, acquaintances, or strangers plays a role in our microbiome. It is absolutely absurd to think that other people could affect your gut health, but that is how things work.

Something such as kissing your partner means that you are sharing your microbes. Your mouth is full of microbes including the teeth, gums, tonsils, and tongue. We are not saying that you should stop sharing your love for your partner because essentially, your mixed microbes are harmless and will help build up healthy microbiomes.

In recent times, it has been drummed into us that we should wash our hands and sanitize frequently because of a potentially deadly virus that is doing the rounds. Not everyone will be affected the same, and you could be one of the lucky ones to escape the virus with just a sniffle. You would have to give your gut microbiome an extra healthy treat as a sign of appreciation.

In order for your microbiome to be as healthy as possible, you need to take care of yourself. Scientists are not able to do that for you. Doctors can offer advice and tell you to take various supplements to ensure a stronger and healthy microbiome. At the end of the day, it is up to you to decide what you want to put into your body and the lifestyle you lead. Again, nobody is going to tell you to stop taking medication prescribed by a medical professional. If your doctor has told you that you need medication, you should follow the advice of your doctor.

In Summary

What have we learned so far about the healthy gut microbiome? Well, we know that the scientists do not have all the answers at their fingertips just yet. We won't hold this against them because we know that they are working as hard as they can to piece all the trillions of pieces of the puzzle together. This could happen in a day, a week, a month, a year, or many years from now. We shouldn't be too hard on the researchers and scientists because we know that they are hard at work trying to figure out a lot of what happens in our bodies.

We know that everything that happens in our bodies is related to our microbiome, which is a community of microbes in our intestines. These gut-healthy critters, known as bacteria, fungi, and viruses, ensure that we are able to live a healthy life. They are ever-growing and changing to fit into our busy lifestyles.

Our very own personalized community living within the confines of our intestines works overtime to ward off any potentially harmful bacteria. They help digest everything we consume, send the nutrients off to the necessary cells and organs to strengthen them, and thus ensure that we live to see another day.

Chapter 2: Unhealthy Gut Microbiome

You have been introduced to the wonderful and mystical world of what happens in the confines of our bodies. You have a better knowledge of how the microbiome works in your intestines to keep you healthy. We know that investigating the microbiome that lives within us is research in progress and scientists are constantly testing new microbes to develop different treatments. In this chapter, we will be looking at the negative side of having an unhealthy microbiome.

Although our bodies have trillions of microbes protecting our intestines and organs by warding off unwanted visitors, harmful bacteria do slip through the cracks. These harmful bacteria are known as pathogens.

They can enter our bodies in various ways such as through the mouth, open wounds, eyes, or nose. The pathogens are spread via contact with others, airborne droplets spread by sneezing or coughing, or body fluids. Indirect spreading includes doorknobs, countertops, shopping carts, or flushing the toilet. There are many ways in which pathogens can enter our bodies to cause a variety of illnesses and diseases.

In order to proceed with the next steps of protecting our bodies from illness, we need to look at the possible issues that can affect your overall health and well-being. We are going to look at some of the possible causes that affect people who have a compromised or unhealthy gut microbiome. This is not to say that everyone will have the same experiences or symptoms. The severity of illnesses and viruses vary from person to person due to their microbe makeup.

Stomach Issues

This is probably one of the most common signs of a compromised gut microbiome. Everything happens in our stomachs. Whatever we consume settles in our intestines. Our army of microbes works overtime to help process and digest what we take in. If your microbiome is unhealthy, you can experience various issues such as constipation, diarrhea, bloating, or heartburn. We have all experienced these issues at some point in our lives. These can occur due to not eating the right amount of dietary fiber or foods that irritate our stomachs, which could be anything from bread to bananas or spices.

Determining what you can and cannot eat, or what you should and not eat, is a process of trial and error. You might love tomatoes, but one bite could mean your stomach does not agree with your love. You will feel the heartburn or cramps almost instantly. It could be that your gut microbiome is not adequately equipped to deal with the acid.

Similarly, you might love eating everything related to strawberries. You have no issues eating fresh strawberries, but the moment you drink a strawberry milkshake or eat strawberry yogurt, you can feel your stomach churning. It could be that your gut microbiome, which tolerates dairy, does not like the combination of the two.

We will take a look at a couple of stomach-related issues that are slightly more severe and cause us discomfort. There are many causes ranging from stress and diet to the lifestyle we lead. How you incorporate the necessary changes to ensure your comfort and well-being are up to you.

Irritable Bowel Syndrome (IBS)

This is one of the most common stomach related issues that exist. It can affect everyone at some point in their lives. Irritable bowel syndrome is an issue that can be classified as a chronic condition. The symptoms mimic those of normal stomach issues such as constipation, diarrhea, cramping, severe abdominal pain, and/or blood in the stools. If these symptoms are consistent and causing you discomfort to the point of preventing you from performing your normal daily activities, a trip to your medical practitioner would be strongly recommended.

There could be many causes for your irritable bowel syndrome which range from inflammation in the intestines to how the muscles in your intestines contract, as well as the microflora in your body. This is one way your army of microbes plays an important role in your intestines. New bacteria enter our bodies without us knowing, which is why it is important to take precautions. Pay attention to what you eat and how you feel. Yes, this is easier said than done because you would normally consume something without really thinking. No one can be blamed for the changes in your microbiome, not even you. Stress, hormones, and food all play a role in the changes we experience.

It is how we deal with these changes moving forward that can make a difference.

All hope is not lost when you are diagnosed with irritable bowel syndrome. It is manageable by taking care of what you eat and drink. Start by eliminating certain foods that are known to irritate the gut such as wheat, acidic fruit and vegetables, beans, cabbage, dairy, and sodas. You can also find ways to relieve stress naturally such as reading a book, watching a movie, taking a walk around the neighborhood, or having a relaxing bath. When you have figured out what works best for you in your situation, you will be able to get a handle on your illness.

Crohn's Disease

It is believed that Crohn's disease was diagnosed as far back as 1932 by three doctors, Doctor Burrill Crohn, Doctor Leon Ginzberg, and Doctor Gordon Oppenheimer. When first presented with patients suffering from various stomach issues, including fever and weight loss, it was thought to be tuberculosis in the small intestine. After some research, they discovered that it was an unknown disease that they named ileitis and which later became known as Crohn's disease.

Over the years, extensive research has been done to establish the exact causes and treatments. Research is still ongoing, but for now, Crohn's disease has been determined to be an inflammatory bowel disease. The symptoms associated with this disease are severe cramping in the abdomen, diarrhea, weight loss, malnutrition, and overall exhaustion. If you have abdominal pains, blood in your stools, weight loss, and/or a fever over a couple of days, a visit to your medical practitioner is recommended.

It is believed that Crohn's disease could be in your genes, handed down from family members who have suffered similar ailments.

There is a whole list of possible causes that could also cause you to contract this debilitating disease, such as your age, ethnicity, and smoking. While this might all seem like a death sentence, especially knowing that there is no cure, all hope is not lost. You will be able to manage your condition by taking care of what you eat. It is advisable to cut out fresh fruits and vegetables that could increase your bowel movements, and sorry for caffeine addicts, that is something that should be eliminated too.

During this whole process, your community of microbes is working hard to keep everything balanced, but as we have mentioned previously, those nasty critters slip through the cracks and wreak havoc. Listen to your body and do not ignore the warning bells because you like something. Those alarm sirens go off for a reason, and your microbiome needs a little bit of assistance from you so that they can catch up and repair what is necessary.

Sugar

You've been waiting for this one to crop up, considering that this book is about health and well-being. No one is going to hit you over the head, grab all your candy, and toss it in the trash can. No one ever said you cannot eat a piece of candy or drink sugar in your tea/coffee. We all need a little sweetness in our lives, especially in our current climate where everyone is worried about all the issues of the world. The code word is moderation.

Even though we might be controlling how much sugary treats we consume, there are additional hidden sugars we are not aware of. Those are the sugars we need to take a closer look at because they can destroy our good bacteria and make us susceptible to diseases, and in some instances, even cancer.

Everything that enters our bodies is broken down according to what we eat, where the necessary nutrients are directed, and their purpose in our various cells and organs. Some foods are easier to break down than others. If we were eating only whole foods, we would have a very happy and healthy gut, but this is not the case, unfortunately. Over the centuries, the way our food is processed has changed. In fact, this is something that changes on a daily basis. Due to convenience, we might read a label or two, see the words low sugar, low carb or fat-free, and toss it into our shopping carts.

Reading the fine print on those labels might rock your foundation when you start looking up what some of those additives actually mean. What you thought was healthy, might not be all that healthy after all. Let us take a look at some of the ways our convenience foods have been processed.

Foods

There are many different ways in which the food we purchase at the store has been processed before it reaches our pantries and freezers. The processes involved include food being frozen, canned, baked, pasteurized, and dried. There are various ways in which the foods are processed starting with the simplest, whereby vegetables may be washed, cut, and portioned into packages for resale. Then there are the highly processed foods that are packed with extra sugar, oils, and salt. Before you pick up that next convenience meal or frozen pizza, read the ingredients.

Processed foods are packed with preservatives and additives to extend the shelf life and ensure they are safe for consumption. Now that you know that your convenience foods are filled with preservatives, you can pay closer attention to the ingredients on the packaging such as dextrose, trans fats, and hydrogenated oils. We will take a look at a couple of our favorite foods to see what they can potentially mean to our gut microbiome, in addition to our waistlines.

We have selected a couple of examples to showcase pro-cessed foods and the effects they could have on your bodies. There are many more that you can read up about, foods you thought were healthy because the wrapping or society tells you it is good for your body. If we have to tell you that you shouldn't eat or drink this, that and the other, you are going to do the opposite. You are in control of what you put into your body. Read the labels, look up words you do not recognize, compare them to healthier versions. We are not telling you to stop eating all your favorite foods, but be responsible and use them in moderation.

Bacon

Who can resist bacon? The delicious smell wafting through the house at any given time of the day sends all kinds of happy signals to your brain and stomach. However much we all love the smell and taste of bacon, we have to have a look at what makes it so addictive. You might not be happy with the find-ings, but we need to cover our bases to ensure you have all the necessary information. Bacon is full of salt which can affect our blood pressure. In addition, there are copious amounts of saturated fats and preservatives which can lead to heart dis-ease and obesity.

Flavored Nuts

Nuts are healthy, full of good oils and protein to keep our community of gut microbes happy. Nuts that have been roasted, toasted, and served plain without any additives are good for your body. The problem arises when there are flavor-ings added such as the delicious bar, salted, or candied nuts. These delicious evils are full of sugar, fat, and salt that could lead to a whole range of dietary issues, including dental prob-lems. In order to keep with the healthy gut theme, opt for raw and unprocessed nuts such as cashews, pistachios, almonds, and walnuts.

Microwave Popcorn

You may be feeling despondent as we go through the list of your favorite foods and treats and popping all your happy bubbles. The problem with this favorite study or movie treat is not the popcorn. Standing alone, you can eat popcorn you have popped yourself, but combined with the salt and butter in the bags, that will send your gut microbiome into a frenzy. Researchers have found that the bags of microwave popcorn contain chemicals that can be harmful to your body, causing kidney issues and a whole host of problems. If you want to be in control of how much butter and salt you have in your favorite treat, it is better and healthier to pop those kernels yourself.

Ramen Noodles

This is a firm favorite in most households throughout the whole world. It is a quick and easy meal to prepare in minutes when you have a hungry child screaming in your ear, a busy college student who is cramming for exams, or just want a comfort snack. Ramen noodles have no nutritional values other than a high amount of salt which could lead to high blood pressure. If you want a happy and healthy gut with little to no issues, opt for healthier versions.

Ketchup

This is a condiment that everyone hates to love. The love-hate relationship with ketchup is that it can be used on everything. This is a firm favorite in all households throughout the world. It is used as a dunking sauce for fries and nuggets, or as a tasty sauce for your mouth-watering hamburger. We are about to burst your bubble once again to inform you that ketchup is highly processed. It is jam-packed with sugar and salt, and it has absolutely no nutritional value. You might be better off eating half a cup of sugar with flavoring.

Sleeping Issues

There is absolutely no way my sleeping habits are related to my gut. Wrong! What happens in the gut, affects everything in your body. Let that sink in for a couple of seconds. As children, we were always told that if we do not get enough sleep, we will not grow up properly. The amount of sleep you should get depends on your age, and as you get older, you are able to function on eight hours of sleep.

Some are not that lucky. Yes, they will go to bed at a certain time but they end up tossing and turning the whole night long. No matter how tired you are, your brain just will not stop working and trying to solve next week's problem today. There are normally pretty good reasons why the sandman skips us such as our stress levels, suffering from depression, anxiety, or over-stimulating the brain with too much screen time.

Until now, we have learned that a healthy gut is a happy gut. Research has proven that if we have a flailing digestive system due to an unhealthy diet, our microbiome has to work overtime to break everything down and send it to the correct departments. Lack of sleep, increased/decreased appetite, and obesity are in cahoots with each other, thus influencing the gut microbiome.

Studies have proven that if you are sleep deprived, it can affect your appetite making you more inclined to snack on unhealthy treats like ramen noodles or inhale a tub of ice cream. In other words, if you are sleep deprived and snacking, you could gain weight. Sleep deprivation affects the production of leptin, which is one of the hormones from our fat cells, which prevents it from telling the brain that it doesn't need food. This is just one example of how our gut microbiome is able to affect our sleep patterns, as well as our cognitive thinking.

Lack of sleep can almost certainly affect your mood. There is nothing worse than taking out your frustrations on an innocent bystander because you didn't get enough sleep.

Try eating a light meal in the evenings. If you implement one little change, you could be helping your hard-working army process and break down everything quicker. This could mean that by the time you go to bed, your body will be peaceful so that you can relax and fall asleep with ease.

As previously mentioned, scientists are constantly researching the microbiome and the effects it has on the rest of our bodies. One thing is certain, we have learned that what we consume affects just about everything in our bodies. It is an eye-opener to realize, after discovering you have bacteria living inside your body, how everything is working. You might even be learning how to respect your body a bit more.

In Summary

This chapter has been an emotional rollercoaster of discoveries. What have you taken away from this chapter? Are you still hung up on the fact that bacon is not such a good option, or that your go-to comfort food has no nutritional value? If there is one thing that can be taken away after reading this chapter, it is that you should show your gut microbiome a little bit more respect than you have up till now.

A lot of the issues you struggle with are manageable by a simple tweak here and there. Just exchanging one bad habit with a good one will already shift the gears. The keyword when discussing processed foods was moderation. No one can hold a gun to your head and tell you not to eat or drink this or that. You are capable of making your own decisions. Whatever you decide to do, it will be your decision. You know your body better than anyone else. You know what foods your body can tolerate.

Chapter 3: Improving Your Gut Microbiome

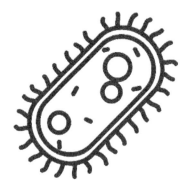

66 Don't put off until tomorrow what you can do today" is an excellent piece of advice given by Benjamin Franklin, one of the Founding Fathers of the United States. We all procrastinate, it is human nature to want to do something later, tomorrow, or next week. This is something every human being is guilty of, and if you have never procrastinated, please be sure to share how you have done that.

All jokes aside, we do tend to put off starting something and as the starting time or date draws closer, we find ways to work around it thus delaying the process even more. This will apply to all aspects of our lives.

You know in your gut that you need to work on your health by eating healthily, exercising, stopping smoking, or getting sufficient rest. Monday or New Year's resolutions are the most common starting days for any major changes in our lives. Every day should be a Monday, there is no time like the present to start caring for yourself.

Make little changes at first. Map out your strategies. Make a list of what you would like to accomplish. Remember, your microbiome has been working for you since the day you came into this world. Now is the time to start helping your community of microbes cope with new and improved threats that enter your body on a daily basis. We know just about all we need to know about airborne viruses and harmful bacteria. We have learned that these nasty pathogens can affect us in many ways, but we tend to turn a blind eye and say, "I am healthy, I won't get sick."

Never say never. We know that no matter how healthy we are, harmful bacteria will enter our bodies and can slip through the cracks. You do not want to be sick. It is not nice having a sore body, sniffles, and coughs. By taking care of yourself and what you put into your mouth, you are already minimizing any possible attacks. Let us take a look at ways in which we can improve our gut microbiome. These will not break the bank, and we will not send you off to the health food store to stock up on supplements. We are going to be doing this naturally and holistically. This is not a quick fix, but rather a long-term mechanical tune-up. Keep in mind that not all the foods we will be talking about in this chapter will agree with everyone. This is a topic we will be discussing further in the book. This is merely a guideline showcasing what could be used as alternatives to medication.

Restoring Gut Flora

The army of bacteria in our intestines is important to our bodies. When the intestines are unhappy, it can lead to various problems that could affect your overall well-being. In order to help protect and build up your army, you need to supplement your body with probiotics. We have all heard about probiotics. Many doctors and healthcare advisors advise taking probiotics when you are taking antibiotics for infections. We are going to look at a variety of probiotic-enriched foods that could be implemented into our diets.

Dairy Products

Many have a love-hate relationship with cottage cheese. It could be the texture, either coarse or smooth, or it could be the strong taste. No one is going to tell you to eat it by the spoonful, but a helping a day could make all the difference your gut might need to heal and repair itself. Cottage cheese contains live and active cultures that help the microbiome in their battle to ward off unhealthy bacteria. As an added bonus, cottage cheese is high in calcium which is good for your bones and teeth.

Parmesan cheese, which is a fermented cheese that contains lactic acid bacteria, is another good option. Parmesan cheese is commonly associated with pasta and pizza dishes but is also an ideal snack option when sprinkled over popcorn or eaten as is. This rich cheese contains protein and calcium.

Plain yogurts are rich in probiotics that will help strengthen your digestive system and protect it against harmful entities. If you have a hard time swallowing plain, unflavored yogurt, consider adding fruit, plain nuts, and seeds.

We recommend eating yogurt cold, as when it is warmed or incorporated into cooked meals, it will kill off the live cultures that are so important to our digestive systems.

Fermented Vegetables

You can buy or make your own fermented vegetables but take careful note of the preservatives used. What exactly are fermented vegetables? The whole process is fascinating, as you will be converting carbohydrates into organic acids using the microorganisms in the produce. You will be growing healthy bacteria to strengthen your gut microbiome.

The vegetables are fermented by using vinegar or brine water. In order for the fermented vegetables to perform their tasks efficiently within your intestines, you will need to ensure that you choose the brine solution which is a natural process. Fermented foods such as cucumbers, cabbage, onions, or carrots can be incorporated in salads or eaten as is. It is not advisable to warm or incorporate your preserved vegetables into cooked meals as it will affect the healthy bacteria.

Naturally Increasing Good Bacteria

By now we know that maintaining our gut microbiome is important to our health. We have to take care of what we eat and introduce a variety of unprocessed foods. In modern times, this is not always possible due to the ever-changing world we live in. Food has always been a part of our lives, since the beginning of time. To keep up with the changing times, producers and manufacturers have had to find ways in which to make the process of living easier. In doing this, they have found ways that would be convenient for us to spend less time on preparing nutritious meals and more time being productive in the workplace.

We need to start taking care of ourselves. We want to be able to live a long and healthy life without succumbing to the medical threats of the world. In order to do this, we need to make some changes. We will have to start taking note of what we eat. Yes, we have said this many times but in order to have this become a reality, we need to stress the importance of a clean and healthy way of life. While probiotics have taught us that it will strengthen and balance our digestive systems, we also need to fill up on healthy dietary fibers which are known as prebiotics.

What in the name of food are prebiotics? Your army of bacteria needs these prebiotics to fuel the probiotics so that they can fight even harder to keep you healthy. You are in control of your diet, so instead of stocking up on canned, packaged and processed foods, opt for whole foods, and prepare them yourself. You can control what you add to your food. Who knows, the way you prepare your food compared to the way the stores sell them might make your children prefer your home-cooked meals and have them coming back for more. Again, no one is telling you that you cannot eat processed foods, but enjoy them as a treat once in a while. Get back to the basics.

Some foods which are full of dietary fiber are rye, whole grains, apples, mushrooms, garlic, carrots, onions, wheat, and legumes. While there are still many more that could be added to this list, you can cook up a delicious meal of healthy fibers using just these. Your microbiome will thank you because you have possibly protected your gut lining or prevented a flare-up of inflammation.

Exercise

Here is another trigger word you were waiting for to appear, the exercise part. You are thinking we are going to make you sign up at the gym for a membership you will probably only use for about two months before the novelty wears off. Hold your horse and cart, because no one is going to make you sign up for anything. You do not need a gym membership. You do not even need exercise equipment at home. All you are going to need is about 30-minutes of your time a day.

The options available to you are easy and simple, and you can do it in the comfort of your home. If and when you feel that you are ready to take the next step, the sky's the limit. It is bizarre to think that exercise can improve your gut health but if you think about it, the more you jiggle and jive, the more you get your insides to move around. At the end of the day, think about your community of microbes having a dance party instead of constantly working on breaking down everything you consume.

Some of the exercises you could try are walking around the neighborhood, jogging, vacuuming your house, running around the garden with the dogs, dancing, and so much more. You can do whatever you feel you want to do, as long as you get moving more. If you can, add in some strengthening exercises, they will also help. Again, you can make do with what you have in your home, such as tinned cans, filling an empty milk container with water, carrying around a pack of flour – improvise and make it fun for yourself. The reason why many people give up on exercising is that they feel intimidated by trying to stick to whatever plans they've made. As a beginner, you do not need a schedule. Dedicate 30 minutes of your day to doing something active. Your microbiome will thank you, and you will feel accomplished about yourself.

Intermittent Fasting

This is something that has been trending in recent years. Everyone seems to be jumping on the intermittent fasting train. There are a lot of misconceptions around fasting. When you mention that you are fasting, people automatically think it is for religious reasons. It has taken celebrities and a focus on various types of diets to put intermittent fasting in the spotlight.

The idea of intermittent fasting is not to starve yourself, or sit staring at the clock and wishing it would tick faster so that you can eat your next meal. Simply explained, intermittent fasting is likened to you having a solid night's sleep without interruption. You are shaking your head because that sounds impossible. Nothing is impossible if you want it enough.

Intermittent fasting is a great way to give your microbiome a break from digesting food all day long. If you give your gut a break from working 24 hours a day, you are helping your body heal from all the activity. Your body, like you, needs a break so that it can be revitalized and energized to fight all the harmful bacteria. In addition, intermittent fasting will help strengthen your gut lining by limiting abrasive activity.

You will not be starving during this time. For at least eight hours, you should be sleeping and if you are not, there are a few tips to help you get through those dark hours while you are pining for the leftover lasagna or the Oreo double-stuffed cookies in the pantry. Ensure that your last meal of the day is filled with protein, healthy fats, and unprocessed carbohydrates such as vegetables. This meal is gut-healthy and will almost definitely tide you over for at least 12 hours.

The trick is to ignore the temptations. That little voice in your head telling you to have a treat, that one will not do anything to you. Resist the temptation, and have a glass of water or a cup of unsweetened black tea or coffee.

If you are not ready to end the day, do something to distract your mind from thinking about food. You are not depriving yourself of anything because you have had a wholesome meal. Listen to some relaxing music. Read a book. Play a game.

When food has ruled your life for a long time and you start taking back control, you will be faced with resistance, but it is your body and you are in control of it. Think about what you want to achieve in the long run. You want to be around to roll around the lounge floor with your children, or you want to be able to live a long and prosperous life. It is achievable. It is not a dream that has to fade away.

Alcohol

We have said it from the start and we will probably continue saying it until the end, no one is forcing you to do anything you do not want to do. We are pointing out ways in which you can improve your gut microbiome to ensure you have a long and healthy life. By having all the advantages and disadvantages of your lifestyle before you, you alone can make the choices. It is entirely up to you.

Have you ever noticed that when you are out with your friends and having a jolly time, each sip you take of your alcoholic beverage causes a burning sensation as it travels down your throat, flows through your chest, and splashes into your stomach? Imagine how your intestines must be feeling. That burning sensation irritates your intestines and lowers the resistance of your microbiome. This lowered resistance could be what harmful bacteria have been waiting for, as they won't have a welcoming committee to give them a scrub down. Even more concerning is that once the alcohol is in your system, it wants to make an exit and will take no hostages.

The last thing you will want in the morning is a stomach full of harmful bacteria because your already healthy bacteria are slightly inebriated and have been prevented from performing their job effectively. You will almost definitely wake up with a hearty headache, in addition to an irritated gut which can lead to diarrhea, excessive gas, and nausea. Looking at this picture, you get an idea of how hard your microbiome works to get rid of harmful bacteria.

If you want to have a drink, consider eating a probiotic-enriched product such as yogurt or a couple of crackers with cottage cheese before you head out the door. Avoid foods prepared in saturated fats. Think about your body and the possible harm you could be inflicting on it. A glass of red wine on occasion is a good option, as it has antioxidants that can help the healthy army of bacteria.

Quick Fix Diets

There is no such thing as a quick fix. As much as we would like to lose those unwanted pounds overnight, it is impossible to achieve this. No matter what the advertisements or ambassadors say, there is no overnight solution. Advertisers are very sneaky when introducing all the shakes, pills, and potions to promote their products. These could set you back a few hundred dollars a month because they use photos of your favorite celebrities to sway your decision.

We are here to pop your bubble once more with the news that there are no magical pills and potions. Fad diets are just that: they might work for a month or so, or until you realize you are being restricted by not eating normal food. This is the same for the diets that are designed to tell you to eliminate all the healthy food your body needs and craves. By depriving your body of the actual nutrients, proteins, healthy fats, and dietary fiber, it will send you running off to the closest McDonald's to fill up on Big Macs, fries, and sugary soda.

Fad diets upset your microbiome, as it is struggling to keep up with whatever you are ingesting. What worked on the mice while researching the products cannot be likened to what is happening in the human microbiome. Two different species leading two separate lifestyles, so to speak. The only way to ensure you have a healthy microbiome and maintain it is to change your lifestyle. A simple lifestyle change is all it will take, and we will be looking at some lifestyle plans to suit every person's dietary requirements. No pills and potions are needed if you make some changes.

In Summary

This was an interesting look at ways in which we can turn negatives into positives. We are slowly moving along and understanding the significance of a healthy lifestyle. By changing this and adopting beneficial habits, you can alter your health in so many ways. There are many ways we can enhance our microbiome which have not been mentioned. You have been presented with some of the most common ways to implement changes.

You have learned that it doesn't take that much effort to keep your community of microbes happy. What they are asking you for is not unreasonable. They just want what is best for you, so that you can lead a healthy life. If you can help your gut, you are helping yourself.

Chapter 4:
The Importance of a
Healthy Lifestyle

We have learned and are still learning how our microbiome works. In order for the healthy bacteria and fungi, our very one personalized army living within the confines of our intestines, to fight for our rights, we need to improve our lifestyle. It is up to each and every one of us to ensure we take care of our own critters. It is almost like having our first pet as a child. It was our responsibility to care for them, keep their cages or bowls clean, and make sure that they were happy at all times. This is how we should live our lives.

We only have one body, and it is up to each individual to ensure that we take care of it.

Living a healthy lifestyle is no easy task. There are so many temptations around us. Every day a new temptation joins the party. You can bet your last dollar that no one has lived a healthy lifestyle since the day they arrived on the earth. Everyone has a second, third, or multiple chances to correct their current lifestyle. It is never too late to change how you live until you have reached your expiry date. Start today, and make little changes at first. It might seem like you are climbing a mountain, but if you persevere, you will feel good about yourself and you will know that you are capable of so much more.

In this chapter, we will be looking into the importance of a healthy lifestyle. There will be some repeats of what has been discussed, but it is necessary to put everything into context to drive home the point of how important it is for you and your health. As previously mentioned, no one is going to bully you into doing anything you do not want to do. This is your choice and you will not be judged. You will need to adopt the same principle by not judging someone who does not look like the poster child of a healthy lifestyle. If you are slender, do not judge or bully people who are more padded. You are just doing what we have promised we wouldn't do to you, and that is bullying and judging. You do not know what their circumstances are. Focus on yourself before you point out others. This book is your personal guide to a healthier you. In this moment, this book is speaking to you and not to your partner – he/she will have to get their own because we are talking to you.

Benefits of a Healthy Lifestyle

You have heard it all. You have done some of your own research. You have seen advertisements promising that you will lose 25 pounds overnight by drinking some or other magic pill.

No matter what you have read or seen, there are no quick fixes. You simply cannot snap your fingers and expect changes in an instant. In order to have and live a healthy lifestyle, you must start with you and how you want to feel.

If you feel you do not need any changes, then so be it, but by picking up this book, something in you was triggered. If you were hoping for a miracle to happen overnight, sorry again, because this is not a fairytale. This is reality and a chance to shift your mindset.

Taking the first steps are scary. Picture the look of a baby learning to take his first steps. The look of fear as he stands up, wobbles around unsteadily, and plops down. His cheering section is giving him the courage to try again. Mom helps him up, steadies him and as he takes his first step, he plops down again. This is something that will keep on happening, but he is growing in confidence as his cheering section offers words of encouragement. It happens, he takes one step, a slight wobble, steadies himself and takes another step into the arms of his supporters. How exciting is this? Baby didn't give up. He stuck it out, and after many unsteady wobbles and falls, he made it to the other side.

Now change the scenario and picture yourself trying something new: your cheering section, which is your microbiome, is celebrating. You have initiated the first steps and your gut is rejoicing because it knows what your intentions are. After stumbles and falls, you too will make the positive changes that are needed for yourself. You have to want this! It is your body and you are in charge of it.

Changing Habits

Simple changes can make all the difference. Instead of having your normal burger, fries, and soda for lunch every day, consider changing things up a few days a week.

Wake up half an hour earlier in the morning and make yourself a turkey, cheese, and tomato on sourdough bread sandwich for lunch. You could also make extra food at night and portion some out in a container to take to work the next day.

Think about the money you will be saving if you skip the drive through a couple of times a week. While you are making your own lunch, add a couple of healthy snacks such as nuts and fruit instead of accosting the vending machine. There are many ways that you can make subtle changes. Over time, these changes will be what you long for and what your body yearns for.

Stop Smoking

This is a habit that many people, no matter where in the world they are, struggle with. It is smelly, it leaves stains on your teeth and fingers, and it can make you ill. We all know that smoking is bad for us. It does not only influence our health, but also those who are around us. What kind of an effect does this smelly habit have on our microbiome? Smoking can change the way your army of bacteria performs their task. If the bacteria cannot perform their task to the best of their ability, they will be letting the bad bacteria filter through. There are a lot of different illnesses and diseases which are related to smoking such as asthma, inflammation in the bowel, as well as lung and colon cancer.

We all know that this is a nasty habit, and you probably have everyone and his/her aunt on your case about quitting. The more you are told you need to stop, the more you light up and puff away. You are probably scared to put the lighter away. Have you ever asked yourself why you are smoking? Try having an earnest chat with yourself and see what conclusions you come to. Look out for tell-tale keywords.

Stress

When you are feeling overwhelmed or worried, do something productive. Go for a brisk walk around the neighborhood. Find a quiet place wherever you are and meditate. Listen to some relaxing music. Take a relaxing bath.

Think of other ways in which to manage your stress other than lighting up.

Boredom

You know you should be cleaning the house, washing the dishes, or mowing the lawn, but you do not feel like doing anything. You are bored because your friends are doing mundane tasks such as those you should be doing. No one wants to play with you. Find something to do. Put on some loud music and dance like you have never danced before. Bake bread or cook a gourmet meal.

Appetite

This is one example that is used most often. Most people are afraid to give up smoking because it makes them eat more or delve into the junk food. Find a hobby to keep your hands and your mind occupied. Look into creative ways such as adult coloring books, building puzzles, putting Lego sets together, or crocheting. You do not have to exchange one bad habit for another.

The ball is in your court. If you have struggled to give up smoking due to some of the reasons mentioned, or if there are others that have not been mentioned, do not be afraid to change things up. We are also not going to tell you to go cold turkey. Make small changes and cut back gradually. Set your own pace. Remember, you are doing this for your health and not for anyone else. If others want to take credit for you quitting, let them because you will know the truth.

Regular Check-Ups

We live in a world that seems to pass in the blink of an eye. We are so focused on everyone around us that we tend to forget ourselves. We are tireless and just keep on with any and all tasks and forget about the important elephant in the room.

It is hard to remember, but as babies, we had regular check-ups at the pediatrician. Growing up, those pediatrician visits turned into wellness visits where we would be weighed, eyes checked, measurements, and so forth. Somewhere along the line, those wellness visits became obsolete because you felt you were no longer a child.

You will never be too old for wellness checks. These wellness checks could inform you of any potential problems or shifts in your body you were not previously aware of. It is also recommended to have your eyes checked regularly due to how they can be affected when making use of screen time for extended periods. The dentist would love to see you every six months to ensure that you are flossing and taking care of your teeth the way you should.

It is crazy to think that the human body could be likened to a car. Our cars need a service every however many miles where they will run diagnostic checks, replace the oil, clear filters and whatnot. We dare not skip our vehicle's maintenance check-up because we worked really hard to be able to afford our dream car. Why would you neglect your own health? Think of the years of blood, sweat, and tears, not to mention the thousands of dollars it took to feed, clothe, and grow your body. You might think you are healthy and in good shape, but what if?

One Step at a Time

Changes can be intimidating. Oh boy, they are downright scary if we were to be honest. Whether it is moving the television from one side of the room to the other or working at a new workstation, it will take getting used to. There will be resistance, and you will want to go back to the way things were before, but you also know that you have to try new ways and that they will eventually grow on you. The same can be said for changing habits.

You do not need to make a checklist of things you need to change at once. A change that radical could set off all kinds of anxiety triggers that will have you cramming four pieces of chocolate, a packet of Cheetos, and a maple bacon donut into your mouth at once. There is no time period attached to whatever changes you want to adopt. Remember, the most important reason to make changes should be for yourself and not for your employer, friends, family, or partner. The moment you say you are doing it for someone else, you will be scrutinized and judged. Every time you put something into your mouth or do something you should not be doing, you will be ridiculed and possibly met with bullying.

For the sake of your sanity and your mental health, do not put any extra pressure on yourself by announcing your intentions. If you want to break bad habits and introduce new healthy habits, do it for your health and well-being. Think about your community of microbes as well. These poor overworked and underpaid critters really do work harder than you will ever know. At the end of the day, if you respect your gut, you will take care of what you put into your body. It is never too late to make changes, however big or small.

No one is perfect, and you are bound to be tempted to slip into your old ways, and that is okay. Do not beat yourself up too much.

Try your best not to make a habit of slipping up, and instead of just giving up and spending the rest of the day scoffing donuts and shakes, or waffles and cream, grab an apple or a square of cheese. Even better, when you feel temptation creeping up, try and do something to distract yourself. You could always bribe yourself with the promise of a trip to the nail salon, the hairdresser, or going for a spa treatment. However tempted you might be, try to avoid the food reward system. Stick to rewards where you can show off without explaining to anyone why you treated yourself. Think outside the box when thinking up rewards.

Did You Know...

It can take between 18 to 254 days to learn a new habit, and approximately 66 days for it to take a role in your life. How insanely crazy is that? The next time someone tells you to change your ways, refer them to the British Journal of Practice as proof of studies that were performed. It just blows the mind that anyone would think that you can change something with the snap of your fingers. What have we been saying since we started on this journey together? You won't be forced into doing anything you do not want to do. Make little changes. Replace this with that. Do not make all the changes at once.

We also know that the sooner you start making the changes, the sooner you make a step in the right direction and the sooner your community of gut bacteria will be on the right road. At the end of the very long road, your health will come out the winner. Whether it takes 254 days to learn a new habit or 66 days for it to become an automatic routine, you are on the right road.

Personal Care

You are probably wondering what on earth personal care has to do with a healthy lifestyle and the microbiome. Well, if you have missed the fine print since you have picked up this book, we will do a quick refresher. When you were born, you were exposed to trillions of microbes that live in and out of your body. These microbes come together to form an army to protect you. Your very own bodyguards! They might not be gun-wielding bodyguards, but they definitely are body-friendly bodyguards.

Personal care has a direct correlation to your health. It is not to say that you are dirty and that you do not care for yourself, but rather, it refers to doing the little things you take for granted.

We all do things as if we are robots and we do not take notice of what we do, such as brushing our teeth or flossing. It is automatic, taught to us from before we could think for ourselves. Next time you brush your teeth or floss, look at yourself in front of the mirror. Poke some fun at yourself and have a laugh.

Laughing is also part of the personal care routine. Laughter is good for the soul. Put your hands on your stomach when you are laughing. You might just be able to feel your army of microbiomes rolling around as you jiggle them around as if they are jumping on a bouncy castle. Did you have a particularly stressful day where everyone seemed to find fault with everything? Draw yourself a bath, add some fragrant bath bombs, decorate the bathroom with calming scented candles, and relax. You could use your bath time to meditate or pray. This is your time to do whatever you want.

In Summary

We know it is important to take care of ourselves and minimize bad habits. We also know that having someone hitting you over the head with a hammer is never going to work. The only way for you to take things seriously and put positive changes in place is for you to be presented with options. Like countless other people, you do not react well to threats. No one reacts well to threats, at least no one who can think clearly for themselves. No, threatening is a form of bullying, and we have promised that no bullying will be taking place on our watch.

In all honesty, though, this chapter has shown you ways in which you are able to turn a negative into a positive. The changes do not need to take place all at once, unless you are super confident that you will be able to pull it off without backtracking to your old ways. No matter what changes you put into motion, be proud of yourself.

If you have an off day, do not fret about it. Our aim is not to restrict you from anything. Restrictions are definitely a form of threat, telling you that if you do this, then that will happen.

This is a modified lifestyle to benefit you. This lifestyle is tailor-made for you. Remember how we have been saying that no two people are the same? The same is going to apply to which lifestyle plan you decide on. This lifestyle change is going to depend on what your microbiome likes as well. In order to prolong your life so that you can live a long and healthy life, we are going to heal you from the inside out. We will be holding hands as we skip across the river stones to welcome the new and improved you.

Chapter 5: Rebooting Your Microbiome

The time has come to learn how to hit the reset button on your health. We are going to reset our gut microbiome. Make sure that you are ready to commit to this process. Make sure that you are doing this for the right reasons, and that you are not being forced into changing your lifestyle for someone else. If you are being forced, or if you are not ready, you will not succeed with this new venture. You have to be a willing participant.

We have explored the do's and don'ts of what you should be eating in previous chapters, along with getting rest and making sure you incorporate exercise into your daily regime. Whomever you speak to will offer their own bit of advice.

To be truthful, if you have to start searching through Google or any other search platform, you will be left with your mouth hanging open at all the information you are presented with. We do not want you to feel overwhelmed. We do not plan on telling you to go and search and implement. No, we want you to feel like you have someone close to you that will explain what is going to happen or even crack a couple of really bad jokes.

No matter what, this book is supposed to be light-hearted and make you feel comfortable without the pressures of the crazy world. In this day and age, everyone is so serious that even a smile seems to be out of order. Well, in our world, we are going to laugh, we are going to have fun, and if we end up shedding a tear, then we shall shed a couple of tears. If you have managed to fast-forward through the first couple of chapters, you might have missed that laughter is an excellent medical treatment for your microbiome. If you have yourself a hearty belly laugh, your microbiome will be jiggling away and tickling your insides because they are happy that you are happy.

There is another way you can excite your microbiome. We are going to take a look at ways in which to reset/reboot your army of personalized bacteria. A lot of the examples to be shared have been used in previous chapters. Apologies are in order if it seems repetitive, but it is always good to have a little refresher. We want the information to be fresh in your mind as we continue exploring. There are various diets, meal plans, quick fixes, and medications that can be used to start rebuilding your microbiome.

There are many different meal and gut-reset plans to choose from. Instead of overwhelming you with five different plans, we will present you with the most important tips you'll need. You will be able to implement the tips in a custom-made plan to suit your needs. Whatever you decide to do, or whatever actions you decide to implement, take it slowly. Ease yourself into it.

Remember, you do not want to get yourself overwhelmed and set off your anxiety triggers. If you are overwhelmed and anxious, your microbiome will feel it as well, and you will feel a shift in your gut.

Boosting Your Microbiome

There are many tips and tricks on how to boost your microbiome. You will be in control at all times. There is no timeframe on how, what, and when to implement these changes. You are not out to impress anyone. Remember, if you are going to be doing this for someone other than yourself, you are doing this for the wrong reasons. Put yourself on the pedestal and embark on this journey for your health and well-being. At the end of the day, you want to enrich and boost your army of microbes to create a strong and diverse community of critters. By persevering, you will obtain this goal and you will be lowering your chance of potential life-threatening and/or debilitating diseases such as arthritis, colitis, diabetes, and obesity.

Fiber Boost

Increase your daily fiber intake by taking in more than 40 grams per day. The fiber will come from fruit, vegetables, and wholesome grains that are not processed. If you are going to opt for the healthy dietary fiber, you will be reducing your chances of getting heart diseases, foiling the attempts of different cancers, and the biggest bonus of all, losing some unnecessary pounds.

Fruit and Vegetables

Incorporate a variety of fruit and vegetables into your daily regime. If you stick to the same old carrot, cucumber, tomato, and apples, you will become very bored very quickly. When you get bored with the food you eat, you will tend to step off the beaten path and find yourself reaching for something that is not on your new plan. In addition, try and opt for seasonal produce. The selection is more diverse, and your microbiome will have a hearty spread of dietary fiber to break down.

High-Fiber Vegetables

It is said that the fiber content of a vegetable is determined by the darkness in color. The darker it is, the more fiber it has. The more fiber it has, the better it is for your digestive system, which allows the food to be broken down quickly and efficiently. The next time someone insists you eat a normal salad packed with lettuce, tomatoes, cucumber, pickles, and olives, you can pick out the lettuce and add some spinach or Swiss chard to fill up your fiber intake for the day. See, small changes can make a huge difference.

Polyphenols

What in the name of microbiomes are polyphenols? Found in plant-based foods such as seeds, berries, green tea, and olive oil, polyphenols are rich in antioxidants. These micronutrients are like champagne to our community of microbes. It is believed that these polyphenols assist with digestion, maintaining a healthy weight, preventing diabetes, and avoiding cardiovascular diseases.

No Snacking

This might be the toughest of all changes to introduce into a reboot regime. The most important thing to remember is to take it one day at a time. Try and push yourself a little further each day, so that you give your digestive system a break between meals. Fill up a bottle of water, put on the music, and get moving to distract yourself.

Live Microbes

We have covered this previously, where we suggested you incorporate fermented foods into your daily lifestyle. Fermented foods are full of live bacteria which are angels to your gut microbiome. You can make your own foods, or buy them at the health food stores. Be careful when buying your fermented products because you will need to read the labels and ingredients carefully to ensure there are no added sugars and additives which will counteract the health benefits of the fermented products. Stick to unsweetened and unflavored yogurt, kefir, and sauerkraut. The options are endless.

Artificial Sweeteners

There is no balance in the sweetness world. We are told that sugar is bad for us. We are told that artificial sweeteners containing aspartame, sucralose, and saccharin are bad for us. We are left feeling as if the world can just swallow us whole because we are expected to drink unsweetened coffee. Okay, to be fair, we do not really need the sugary sweetness but it is nice, just once or twice a day, to have some sugar in our liquid tar. You might have heard the health warnings related to artificial sweeteners, but we are being honest here, and the warnings are there for a reason. They were not just issued to make our lives miserable.

Artificial sweeteners upset our microbiomes and could lead to diseases such as obesity and diabetes. If you really do need some sweetness in your life, opt for natural sweeteners such as stevia, erythritol, and xylitol. These natural sweeteners come with a warning of their own, as they have laxative tendencies.

Outdoors

We live in a society where technology controls our lives. We tend to spend so much time indoors on various screens such as televisions, cell phones, and computers, that we seem to forget that there is a whole other world outside the four walls of our home. Ditch the screens, put on a pair of comfortable shoes, slather on the sunscreen, and head outdoors. Whether you work in the garden or head off for the nearest hiking trail, take in the beauty and sounds of nature. Being outdoors is known to improve moods which relieves stress and is good for your overall well-being.

Medication

Before you start any new lifestyle program, it is strongly recommended that you visit your medical practitioner. We will not be telling you to stop taking your prescription medi-cation, but we would like to caution you to slow down on the non-prescription medication. Pay close attention to the amount of medication you consume, such as painkillers and antacids. These medications can affect your microbiome in a negative way, causing an upset stomach or eating away at your stomach lining.

Improving Digestion

We have given you various tips on how you can boost and reinforce your microbiome. You are slowly but surely implementing the new changes you have adopted into your lifestyle. You still feel as though you are not doing enough and you are feeling a little out of place. You cannot quite put your finger on what is nagging you. Are you doing enough to ensure you are doing everything you are able to for your digestive system? One thing is for certain, changing your lifestyle and eating correctly is addictive. In order for you to maintain your excitement about being healthy, or at least trying to be healthy, you need to push through. You need to remember the reasons why you wanted to change your lifestyle.

Whether it was to lose a couple of pounds, because you found out that you have food allergies, or because you were diagnosed with something more serious like Crohn's disease, do not give up. Even if you just wanted to change your lifestyle for personal reasons, do not give up. View each day as the start of your journey. Wake up excited to see what you will accomplish. Be excited at what you are able to do. Maintain your enthusiasm. There will be days, not may be days, there definitely will be days when you will want to curl up into a ball with a bag of crisps and Reese's Pieces and flip it to the whole experience. That is okay too. All we are asking of you, before you inhale the crisps and Reese's Pieces, is maybe just have half a handful of each and put the rest away. Remember all the work you have done to get to this point. Imagine that your community of microbes has put on their combat gear because they can tell what is about to descend upon them. These microbes are very clever little bugs because they know what is going to happen before you do. Listen to your gut.

Let us take a look at how we can improve and strengthen our digestive system a little more. There are a couple of interesting tips. They are doable and beneficial. If you do not like the taste of something shared here, do not force yourself to eat or drink it. If you are going to feel like you are forced to do something, you will become despondent and we want you to feel included at all times.

Lemon and Warm Water

If you grew up around the older generation, you might remember someone always saying that you should start off your day with warm water. It seems the scientists agree with their assessment, and that drinking warm water helps stimulate the colon. One would think that drinking cold water would actually shock the digestive system into waking up and working faster, but it actually creates the opposite effect. Drinking warm water helps to break down the food so that it can move out of your body without giving it a chance to find spots to hide away. The debate about warm, room temperature, or cold water is and will be ongoing for many years to come. Each temperature setting has its own benefits, but for the purpose of your digestive system, warm water is the way to go.

If the idea of drinking plain warm water does not settle well with your taste buds, you could always add in a squeeze of fresh lemon juice or a slice of lemon. If you are able to eat the lemon, even better, but a lot of people's taste buds would be protesting. Fresh lemons, which are unprocessed and as natural as can be, are full of vitamin C and dietary fiber. Lemons are also a natural diuretic, which is beneficial to flushing out harmful toxins. The combination of warm water and fresh lemons is an excellent option for the overall well-being of your microbiome, as well as for your digestive health.

Fasting

We touched on intermittent fasting in Chapter 3. This particular lifestyle dates back to 1945 when scientists used mice to study the effect of fasting. As we previously mentioned, there are a lot of misconceptions surrounding intermittent fasting. While it is known that fasting is generally used for religious purposes, not many people knew that it was also beneficial to health and well-being. In the last couple of years, intermittent fasting has gained in popularity due to the exposure from advertisement campaigns and celebrities sharing their "secrets".

The bottom line is, intermittent fasting is beneficial to the health and well-being of humans. It is important to stress that intermittent fasting is not a diet. It is part of a lifestyle. While we are hesitant to speak about diets, it has to be mentioned that intermittent fasting can be incorporated in whatever diet plan you end up deciding will suit your needs best. There are many advantages to incorporating intermittent fasting into your lifestyle. Forget the fact that you could lose some stubborn pounds, there are also the benefits of restoring your microbiome and correcting a variety of other problems.

You know you need to go without eating food for a certain amount of hours per day. There are various ways in which you can approach intermittent fasting and nothing is written in stone. As long as you can go for between eight and 16 hours a day, you are on the right track. Not everyone will be able to achieve the goal of fasting for 16 hours, which is not a huge disaster. Start with an eight-hour a day fast, which essentially is the time you are supposed to be sleeping. The more disciplined you become with fasting, the longer you can stretch your time between meals.

You do not have to worry about being food-deprived. You will not starve. The whole idea of intermittent fasting is to give your digestive system an opportunity to rest, and if needed, to heal.

You can drink fluids such as unsweetened and dairy-free tea/coffee and unflavored water. The moment you chew something and swallow, that will signal the end of your fast. When the time comes to break your fast, opt for a meal featuring protein, healthy fats, and unprocessed carbohydrates. Remember to consult with your medical practitioner before you make any changes to your lifestyle.

Destressing

Stress is a major factor in our lives. No matter how many times we discuss this huge elephant that stares at us from every corner of the room, there is no getting away from it. It is no secret that stress plays a huge factor in our everyday lives. If you say that you do not stress, that you do not have a worry in the world, and that you are the happiest person around – congratulations. You might be the only two-legged person walking around that can lay claim to that title.

It is important that you take care of yourself and your mental health. In order to ensure your microbiome has a reset, implement some necessary changes such as drawing up a sleep schedule. Ensure that you get a solid eight to nine hours of sleep a night. If you find that you are struggling to sleep, persevere. Put on some relaxing music to calm you down, listen to a meditation soundtrack, or practice breathing techniques.

If you are feeling overwhelmed with the pressures of the day, or the circumstances which have been unkind to you, take a walk around the neighborhood. Find alternative ways to let go of your stress. We know that the first place we turn to in times of unrest and worry is the pantry, or we head off to the closest drive-through. We need to learn that we cannot always hide behind food. Hiding behind food is going to throw our microbiome out of tune and we will end up with long-term health issues.

There are many other ways in which we can minimize the

stressful situations in our lives, but we need to know that it is up to each of us to ensure that we take care of what is going into our bodies. No one can dictate to us what we should or should not do. We have presented you with so many options, alternative routes, and short of locking you in a padded cell to make sure you are eating this, that and the other, there is not much else we can do. You are armed with some of the tools you need, and we will continue arming you with more to make sure you are well-equipped.

In Summary

This chapter seems to have highlighted a lot of what has been discussed in previous chapters but on closer inspection, there are quite a few more points added. The whole idea is to show you ways in which you can train your digestive system to cope and deal with new situations. We all know most of what has been mentioned, as we have read them on social media, watched YouTube videos, seen advertisements, and so forth.

This book is not going to paint rosy pictures about how you will lose 100 pounds in a month if you follow this or that diet. That is not realistic. The only way to realistically lose weight and maintain that loss, is by changing the way you live. We have mentioned this over and over, but diets are restrictive. Dieticians will be running around in circles when hearing these views. What you are doing is changing, tweaking, or adding to your lifestyle. This is all about healing your body from the inside out.

Chapter 6: Microbiome Enriched Foods

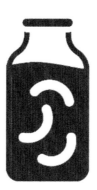

❝ You are what you eat". If taken literally, yes, it is true. After the usual morning coffee infusion, we look like a cup of coffee for the rest of the day. Figuratively speaking, after the first coffee infusion of the day, you feel your intestines wake up as they receive the warm fluid winding its way through your body to its destination. We could spend a couple of chapters describing how each piece of food we eat or beverage we drink works its way through our intestines.

We could think up wild and wonderful stories of how our digestive systems break down the food in a loving way and walk them down the aisle to the next leg of the journey. Yes, that would take more than a couple of chapters to see the love story unfold.

In this chapter, we are going to look into the various types of food categories, and present you with a list of gut-friendly microbiome-enriched foods. It is important that we fill our bodies with antioxidant-rich foods that will protect and nurture our microbiome. We know that we have to help our community of microbes in order for us to be healthy. When you start speaking about how you want to take better care of yourself, the most common words of advice out of people's mouths are to drink supplements or protein-rich shakes. The words of advice get even better when people tell you that you should eat more of this, less of that, and none of those. As previously mentioned, what will work for Joe, does not necessarily word for Mary. You cannot compare your community of microbes to that of your sibling or friend.

We are going to present you with various foods. We have mentioned a few of the foods, but we will be looking at them in a little more detail to see what role they play in our new lifestyle. If you feel uncomfortable adding a certain product to your meal plan, leave it out. If you do not like, say pickles, you do not have to eat it. You do not and will not, be forced to eat anything you do not want to. We are not going to rearrange your taste buds so that you automatically fall in love with something you have never liked before. As we continually have been saying, you are in control at all times.

Probiotics and Prebiotics

Before we look into the food groups, let us take a slight detour from the food map to investigate antibiotics, prebiotics, probiotics. No one is going to tell you not to take prescription medication. If your doctor or healthcare professional prescribes antibiotics or any other medication, you listen to the professionals. If, for some reason you are taking antibiotics, take precautions to protect your gut. Antibiotics are given to patients to combat infections caused by bacteria.

Antibiotics are a necessary evil in order to cure recurring infections such as abscesses, bronchitis, or ear infections. No matter what the illness, your doctor will not prescribe medication you do not need. Yes, antibiotics clear up infections, but they also play nasty games with your microbiome. We are not here to stop you from taking your prescribed medication, but we are here to build up, protect, and strengthen your microbiome. All these "biotics" are intimidating, but each of them presents a different function.

We are going to take a closer look at prebiotics and probiotics. The two should not be confused, as they play different roles in our gut microbiome. There will be a list of foods, and/or beverages that are beneficial and perform specific roles in keeping our intestines, digestive system, and overall well-being churning the way it should be.

Probiotics

What exactly are probiotics? We have already skimmed on, skirted around, or touched on probiotics in a previous chapter. We are going to dive in headfirst into exploring the role probiotics play in our bodies. This is a word you have heard or seen in advertisements, almost all with an image portraying the intestine.

Probiotics are a collection of live bacteria that we ingest in various types of unprocessed, unpasteurized, and natural foods. There are many types of foods that are crammed with healthy gut bacteria which is vital to a healthy body. In order for the foods to perform to the best of their ability, they should not be warmed or heated as it will almost certainly kill off the healthy bacteria that is needed to line your intestines.

Yogurt

Yogurt is a miracle in the limelight. As long as the yogurt is natural, unpasteurized, unprocessed, and unsweetened, you will be lining your intestines with a healthy colony of new bacteria.

Kefir

This delicacy is a fermented milk drink, rich in probiotics. Kefir grains are a combination of lactic acid bacteria and yeast which is added to cow's or goat's milk. Kefir has a number of health benefits such as aiding digestive issues and warding off infections. To add to the benefits of kefir, it can be used by people who are lactose intolerant, as it causes none of the side effects that result from using dairy.

Sauerkraut

This traditional European dish is made from fermented cabbage. Sauerkraut is traditionally served as part of the main meal or as a side dish/salad. In addition to the probiotic qualities, sauerkraut is rich in dietary fiber, vitamins B, C and K, and is high in antioxidants. Make sure you purchase or make unpasteurized sauerkraut. You do not want to lose the health benefits from fermented foods.

Tempeh

Tempeh is a traditional Indonesian product that is made from fermented soybeans. The fermentation process lowers the phytic acid content, but it also produces vitamin B12.

Tempeh is a high-protein product that is rich in probiotics and has a nutty or earthy flavor. Tempeh is an excellent source of protein for anyone wanting to cut down on meat products, including vegans and vegetarians.

Kimchi

Kimchi is a traditional Korean dish made from the main ingredient of cabbage, as well as other vegetables that have gone through the fermentation process. In addition to the vegetable base used, kimchi is flavored with microbiome-friendly seasonings such as red chili flakes, garlic, ginger, and salt. Kimchi is beneficial for your digestive health and is high in vitamins and minerals such as vitamin K, vitamin B2, and iron.

Miso

If you are a fan of cooking shows, you might have noticed that a firm favorite in the pantry that amateur home cooks like to use is miso. Miso is a traditional Japanese soybean seasoning which is used to make soup, as well as flavoring rice and barley. This salty seasoning is made up of fermented soybeans, salt and koji, which is a fungus. Miso is beneficial for your digestive health due to the fiber content, as well as protein. In addition to the nutritional benefits, miso is high in vitamins and minerals.

Prebiotics

After exploring the benefits that probiotics have on our microbiome and overall health, we are going to have a look at the effects of prebiotics. What exactly are prebiotics? We know that probiotics are a collection of live bacteria that we eat or drink to protect our microbiome. Prebiotics are food for your army of bacteria. This food comes from various fibrous carbohydrates that are not easily broken down by the digestive system. The healthy bacteria in your intestines thrive off these different types of fiber.

There are a variety of food types which are beneficial to our microbiome, which we will take a closer look at. Where we were looking at ways to ingest healthy bacteria, we will now be looking at the types of food types used to feed our army of bacteria. The diversity of microbes in our bodies is a game-changer, as there is a constant explosion of new bacteria being cultivated.

Chicory Root

This popular coffee-flavored root is high in fiber known as inulin. The fiber in the chicory root can help your microbiome by relieving constipation and improving digestion, as well are feeding your microbiome. As an added bonus, chicory root aids in weight loss and the antioxidants protect the liver from potential damage.

Dandelion Greens

Wait just a hot minute! Dandelions are weeds that take over our gardens. Correct. They are also nature's gift on a silver platter. This wonderful weed has a whole range of benefits such as reducing constipation, building up the healthy microbiome, and giving the immune system a boost. The benefits do not stop here, dandelion greens are a natural diuretic, they have anti-inflammatory properties, the ability to lower cholesterol, and serve as an antioxidant. When next you are working in the garden and you come across the dandelions, think about what they could mean to your health. They will make an excellent addition to your salad.

Garlic

Who does not like a pizza swimming in garlic, or a delicious garlic bread? Sadly, while this scenario sounds good, the garlic in these two foods is not going to be of benefit to you. As with probiotics, it is best to consume products in their natural state. With garlic, the more you cook and process it, the more of its health benefits it loses. And no, we are not going to tell you to crunch on a clove of garlic.

Unless you want to go to work with a bag over your head to mask the smell, it would be recommended that you use it in salads. The benefits of eating garlic range from reducing the risk of heart disease to alleviating asthmatic symptoms.

Onions

Yes, you are reading between the lines here. You already know the answer to your question. Sorry to say, fried onion rings, while delicious, do not fall in the healthy lifestyle category. You can load up on onions by eating a ton of different salads. Thankfully onions do not smell nearly as lethal as garlic, although they do still have a slight smell that could alert your co-workers that you are on your way. There are a variety of benefits of eating onions such as that it strengthens your microbiome, it aids in breaking down stubborn fat, and it jolts the immune system. The benefits do not stop there, onions also possess antibiotic properties, are an antioxidant, and aid in keeping the cardiovascular system ticking.

Cocoa Beans

Cocoa beans contain flavonoids which are found in plant-based foods such as tea, grapes, and blueberries. When you think of cocoa, your mind automatically associates it with chocolate. If you are a woman, you know that chocolate is your happy food, but you are also realistic that the dream world where chocolate fixes everything is just that – a dream world. No one is ever going to tell you that you can never eat chocolate again. That is a decision only you will be able to make, and again, moderation is key. Cocoa beans are beneficial to the cardiovascular system, as it produces nitric oxide to keep the heart pumping. When broken down, cocoa beans ensure that your army of bacteria are in a happy trance.

Chapter 7: Microbiome-Friendly Food Groups

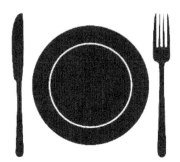

You have been presented with a lot of information over the last five and a half chapters. Some of the information you knew, some you thought you knew but were not too sure of, and some you did not know. In school, you learned about the food pyramid. Over the years, the food pyramid has undergone a transformation. This transformation was necessary to keep up with the ever-changing needs and dietary requirements of the modern world.

We are going to have a look at some of the food groups, which consist of just about everything found in your fridge, freezer, pantry, and garden. Remember that what we will be sharing are guides to what you could use to strengthen, care for, and nurture your microbiome.

In the next chapter, we will be taking a look at some of the lifestyles you can adapt to suit you, and you will be able to incorporate these food groups. While we will only be listing a couple of examples per section, to highlight their properties and what they could mean to your health, you are free to explore and research your favorites.

Vegetables

Love them or hate them, vegetables have been a part of our lives since before we could speak or think. I remember having Sunday lunch at grandma's house, and one of the vegetables that always seemed to be on the menu was carrots, pumpkin, and potatoes. Someone needs to let grandma know that if you eat your pumpkin, you will not get curly hair. She might have been misinformed on some of her old wives' tales, but it was always a treat to listen to grandma's stories and eat her delicious meals.

Vegetables are full of vitamins and minerals which are beneficial to our overall health, but there are some added benefits which is why we are encouraged to eat a variety. We do not eat to eat the same vegetables day after day. If you end up eating a carrot, a piece of broccoli, and a cabbage every day, you will be bored and end up searching for snacks in the unhealthy food group in your mind. Add different vegetables, or at least prepare them differently so that you are not easily turned off.

A word of caution, when you are going to be cooking your vegetables, take care not to overcook them to the point of mush. If you do not care to eat them raw, consider cooking them until they are al dente. If you are unsure what al dente means, a simple explanation is that whatever you make is cooked but still firm when biting into it.

Carrots

Carrots can be eaten in many different ways. You can make fermented carrots, which are soaked in a brine solution for a period of time. You can enjoy carrots raw, as a healthy treat instead of reaching for a bag of crisps. You can incorporate carrots into stews or salads. The sky's the limit where carrots are concerned. Carrots are high in fiber, beta carotene, anti-oxidants, potassium, and vitamin K1. Extra health benefits include lowering the cholesterol levels, and the vitamin A found in carrots helps maintain your vision.

Asparagus

Asparagus is an acquired taste for many. Love it or not, this vegetable can do a lot for your microbiome. Asparagus is also an excellent source of prebiotic fiber which will feed your army of bacteria. You might have heard from someone in passing that if you eat asparagus, you will want to avoid urinating because of the pungent aroma. If you smell it, it is a sign that it is working wonders in your gut, cleansing and doing all that it should be doing. If you are looking for a natural diuretic, asparagus is your best friend. You can roast, boil, grill, or steam your asparagus, drizzle some lemons juice over, a crack of salt, and enjoy it as a snack. If you do not want to snack on asparagus, you can enjoy it as a part of breakfast meals, with pasta, or as a side to your main dish.

Jerusalem Artichoke

Another prebiotic-enriched root vegetable, the Jerusalem artichoke contains a healthy dose of inulin, which is a fiber that balances blood sugar. It is also something that your community of microbes feasts on the way we feast on our favorite treats. The Jerusalem artichoke hails from North America and resembles ginger roots and potatoes. You can enjoy this delicious, earthy root vegetable by roasting, boiling, steaming, or pureeing it. A word of caution, your microbiome will love these vegetables so much, that it will treat you to an aroma of petrified gasses.

Leeks

Leeks fall under the same category as onions, in that they are family. It is a well-known fact that leeks are the emblem for Wales. Even though it is a Welsh vegetable, it is loved by people all around the world. Leeks are also high in inulin, the prebiotic food that keeps your army happy, as well as full of antioxidants to protect the stomach and the colon. You can incorporate leeks into your meals by adding it to stews or making a mouthwatering, stomach-warming potato and leek soup.

Miscellaneous

We can go through all the vegetables, their families, and pick up some stragglers along the way and lump them all together under the vegetable section. There are so many different types of vegetables and each one adds their own unique dynamic to the microbiome. What vegetables have we not mentioned, that we should have mentioned? Brussel sprouts, broccoli, cauliflower, beans, peas, and so many more. You can prepare your vegetables in many different ways such as steaming, boiling, grilling, and fermenting. Vegetables can be enjoyed in soups, stews, salads, or as side dishes. Be creative. The more creative you are, the less bored and predictable you will be.

Grains

This is an interesting food group on the pyramid. Over the years, a lot of doctors, scientists and researchers have weighed in on the grain train. We are not here to force any one specific lifestyle on anyone. We are presenting you with options and many of our own takes on how we perceive things. Everyone is allowed to have an opinion without involving the food police. This is a very delicate food group. How you proceed is entirely up to you. You know your body better than anyone, and you know what it can tolerate.

There are many who can eat copious amounts of grains without any problems, and there are those that can eat a single bite and feel like they are about to float away. No two people have the same experiences.

We are not going to offend anyone from the carbohydrate police. Instead, we are going to carry on and give you some types of grains you can enjoy without feeling guilty. At the end of the day, it is your army of microbiomes you are trying to please, and not that of any know-it-all who is going to tar and feather you for enjoying a slice of sourdough bread. In this book, no one will judge you.

Oatmeal

Oatmeal is a water-soluble fiber that passes through your intestines slowly. The whole idea of food traveling through your body at a snail's pace is to give you the feeling of being sated for longer. Oats contain beta-glucan which is beneficial to lower the cholesterol levels of those with high cholesterol. The most common way to consume oats is by eating it for breakfast. There are other ways in which oats can be used such as in smoothies, baking breads, and making cookies.

Oat Bran

What is the difference between oatmeal and oat bran? They are very similar in that they are both water-soluble fiber and they both contain beta-glucan. Oat bran is beneficial in improving blood sugar levels and regulating blood pressure. Oat bran is added to smoothies, muffin mixes, and bread dough. One of the benefits of this fiber-rich grain is that it helps in keeping the intestines churning so that everything will ebb and flow the way it should be.

Quinoa

This miracle grain has been around for centuries. It is high in fiber, iron, potassium, calcium, magnesium, and a whole lot of other wonderful nutrients.

The best part is that quinoa is gluten-free. Hailing from South America, this grain can be found in white, red, and black varieties. There is nothing bad to say about these little pieces of golden grain. Quinoa is prepared as if you are cooking rice, add a crack of salt, and enjoy your guilt-free meal addition.

Buckwheat

This whole grain is filled with protein and fiber, as well as helping to manage diabetes and aid in weight loss. Buckwheat and quinoa seem to be family, as both have similar nutritional benefits. We have to mention that care should be taken in case you suffer from an allergy. All foods should be treated with caution, especially when you are introducing new foods. If you are experiencing symptoms such as swelling of the tongue or breaking out in hives, please take your allergy medication. Buckwheat can be used as a breakfast food, incorporated into a salad for lunch, added to stir-fry as a filler, or used to make a gluten-free muffin for dessert.

Miscellaneous

There are many different types of grains we can cover. The anti-carbohydrate police are going to be breaking down doors because we are not going to succumb to their bullying tactics. If you want to eat rice, go ahead and eat the rice, or if you want a baked potato, go and enjoy your baked potato. We have consistently said that moderation is the takeaway through every lifestyle change. Whatever you decide to put into your body, listen to your gut. If your gut says that it has had enough, do not push it further than its limits. The more you eat, the harder your digestive system has to work.

Fruit

Who does not like fruit? If you walk around the shopping mall and munch on something that could have been a little healthier, you will get the odd person that will pass a snide comment that you should rather eat fruit. This type of comment is very hurtful, especially when you know you are tipping the scales a little more than you should. People shouldn't be allowed to pass judgment. Whatever the case, you have been not so subtly told you should eat fruit instead. Okay, so we will look at the fruit in the fresh produce aisle at the grocery store.

There are lots of different fruits. It is really amusing how people can say why you should be eating fruit, but as with all other types of food, no one knows if you have a particular intolerance to that food. Danny loves oranges. He can eat three oranges in one sitting. As much as he loves oranges, it is not to say that those oranges are returning the love. Every piece of food that is out in the world is not going to have the same effect on each person. Poor Danny is in agony by the time he has finished his oranges. His intestines are protesting as if they've lost the battle of the bands. Why does this happen?

Oranges

While we are using the orange scenario and Danny's intestines, we will take a look at what this is about. Oranges are high in vitamin C which boosts the immune system against colds and certain infections, as well as preventing skin damage, lowering cholesterol, blood pressure, and the risk of cancer. There is nothing bad about oranges because all that we can see right now is all the wonderful benefits, including that it is high in fiber. We all know how our army of microbes love additional fiber. Why were Danny's intestines having all kinds of meltdowns? In short, he was making a pig of himself and the high fiber was not being all that friendly. An orange a day should be good. Remember, fresh is best. If you want orange juice, bring out the juicer to make your own.

Store-bought juice, even when it says it is 100%, still has additives. If you want optimal benefits, stick to the real fruit.

Bananas

High in soluble and insoluble fiber, bananas are one of your intestines' best party fruits. Bananas can be incorporated into your oatmeal breakfast, a smoothie, sliced up in yogurt, or eaten au natural. Now because you get excited, we are not talking about baking banana breads and including that in your diet. We are talking about the whole fruit, eaten as it was intended. Bananas can keep your feeling fuller for longer, which would be an ideal way to kickstart your intermittent fasting. Bananas are full of delicious nutrients such as potassium, calcium, vitamin B6, iron, and many more. When next you are tempted to indulge in the banana muffin at Starbucks, or the freshly baked loaf in your kitchen, stop, take a step back, and retrace your steps to the fruit aisle at the grocery store and pick up a bunch of fresh bananas instead.

Apples

Apples awaken all kinds of happy triggers in the intestines. As with bananas and oranges, apples are high in soluble fiber and water. It is advisable to munch on your apple with the skin still on, as all the nutrients are found in the skin. The health benefits of the crunchy apple include lowering cholesterol levels, providing a rich variety of antioxidants, lowering blood pressure, and the added bonus of weight loss. Your army of good bacteria will be very happy if you give them an apple a day, as the pectin, which is the fiber in the apple, is an excellent prebiotic. If you have ever wondered whether the saying "an apple a day, keeps the doctor away" is true, you can stop wondering, as it is true. Apples have many healing and prevention capabilities against diabetes, cancers, protect your stomach against certain medications, as well as stimulating the brain.

Berries

If you do not include berries in your daily meal plan, you are missing out. Berries are rich in antioxidants, are likely to improve blood sugar levels, and contain soluble fiber to ensure you feel sated for longer periods of time. Adding berries to your breakfast oatmeal or smoothie is also a great way to get the beneficial nutrients your body can thrive on. There are a variety of berries such as strawberries, blueberries, blackberries, youngberries, and raspberries. These nutrient-rich fruits can be added to smoothies, yogurt, oatmeal, or fruit salads. There is no limit to your creativity. The health benefits in berries are endless, ranging from being good for your skin and lowering cholesterol levels to protecting you against possible cancers.

Miscellaneous

Fruits have become a firm favorite of the food pyramid. Without having any of the aforementioned fruits around, you envision what they would smell and taste like. This trickery is teasing all the senses of your stomach to wake up and poke you deep from within to say that this is what they want, what they are demanding. We have already mentioned that fresh is best. If at all possible, steer clear of processed fruits, which are more often than not laden with syrups, extra sugar, and cooked until all the goodness has been killed off. There are tons of different fruits that offer excellent beneficial health properties such as pineapples which help for inflammation, avocados which are good for the heart and digestion, and tomatoes which are rich in vitamin C, antioxidants, vitamin K, and potassium. You will never go wrong with fresh fruit. Each season will present you with the best seasonal fruit to benefit your health and well-being.

Dairy

In Chapter 3, we spoke about the various dairy products that would benefit your army of microbes. We focused on all the live cultures that would send in new bacteria to befriend those already living there and to help them gain in strength. Dairy is a very tricky part of everyone's diet. Many people suffer from lactose intolerance which affects their intestines and sends them on a wild roller coaster ride. At each turn, something will come to the surface such as rashes, cramping, nausea, and inflammation.

To gain the optimum health benefits from dairy products, be selective and know what you are putting into your body. We have learned so far that we need to lay off the processed goods, as they have been manipulated and depleted of all the good nutrients. In this section, we will continue placing our focus on the natural dairy products. Know what you are getting and what you are putting into your body. We are most certainly not going to tell you not ever to drink this milk or eat that cheese. No, there will be none of that. At the end of the day, we all want to be healthier and do what we can do to make sure we achieve that goal.

Since we have spoken about the various dairy products, this section will be short. There is no need for a refresher course in the dairy department. Read the labels, know what to look for, know what to avoid and follow your gut instinct. You can incorporate what you have learned in the previous chapters into your new lifestyle.

Fats

This is yet another controversial topic in the land of lifestyles. There are so many different types of diets that say, yes, incorporate high-fat foods into your new lifestyle. There are those that say no, high-carb and low-fat diets are the way to go. This is going to end up in a tug of war between all the millions of diets/lifestyles that are floating around the wonderful world wide web, or individualized personal diets. This is a train that will be going around in endless circles because everyone will be confused. We are of the opinion that we will leave the decision to you, the reader, what you would like to do once we have a look at some of the lifestyles in the next chapter. You are an adult and you are more than capable of making the decision for yourself.

After a bit of a giggle while trying to decipher what types of fats would be considered healthy, a return search gave no information other than to say that all fat is bad and should be avoided. It is astounding how, one can almost say, narrow-minded, the so-called health nuts really are. If it were up to them, every single person who is eating sweet potato fries that have been fried using coconut oil is joining the obesity club. This is just the opinion of someone who has been through enough regimented diets, diet clubs, and quick fixes to spot these things like a glaring pimple on a small nose. In all seriousness, if you were told to avoid this, that, and the other, you would be eating nothing but soil and fresh air.

Extra Virgin Olive Oil

Olive oil is made from the fruit of the olive tree. The fruit being that little green blob you get in your martini. There are two types of olive oil; extra virgin olive oil is made from cold-pressed olives, while the regular olive oil is a blend of processed and cold-pressed oils. Extra virgin olive oil is rich in monounsaturated oleic acid and antioxidants.

The health benefits include being an anti-inflammatory ambassador which will fight type 2 diabetes, arthritis, cardiovascular disease, and Alzheimer's. Extra virgin olive oil is not linked to weight gain or obesity and has antibacterial properties. The bottom line is, extra virgin olive oil is good for you and your microbiome. You can fry your steak or fish, or you can make up a salad dressing and enjoy a guilt-free oil that promises only healthy properties.

Sunflower Oil

According to various lifestyle plans, sunflower oil is persona non grata. Yet, according to researchers who spend their time looking into the scientific evidence, sunflower oil is beneficial to our health and well-being. Sunflower oil is high in monounsaturated fats which are good for the heart. To add to the benefits, it is rich in vitamins A and E which ensure your skin will glow, as the vitamins are high in antioxidants. Sunflower oil will also help with your digestions, as it has laxative tendencies which can help alleviate constipation. As an added benefit, sunflower oils can be used for personal care routines such as massaging it into your skin and as a conditioner to tame frizzy and dry hair.

Coconut Oil

Coconut oil is high in saturated fats and is beneficial to your health, and it will aid in weight loss, assist with brain fog, and promote a healthy heart. The medium-chain triglycerides in coconut oil are full of amazing healing benefits such as using it as a mouthwash, curbing appetites, and raising the levels of good cholesterol. As if the health and healing benefits were not enough, coconut oil can be used for personal care such as moisturizing the skin, protecting your skin from damage, and taming out of control hair. To make sure that you get the best coconut oil, ensure that you steer clear of the refined and processed ones, and rather opt for the organic and unprocessed kinds.

Grass-Fed Butter

There was a little bit of hemming and hawing about which section this butter should go in, but since it is related to the fat part of the food pyramid, it is going to remain right here. Butter is made from cow's milk. Grass-fed butter is more nutritious than normal butter, as it has more healthy unsaturated fatty acids such as omega 3 fatty acids, as well as a healthy dose of vitamins K2 and A. Regular butter does not contain nearly the same amount of healthy antioxidants as grass-fed butter. The bottom line is, when you cook with grass-fed butter, your food will have a rich flavor that you cannot get from oil, regular butter, or margarine.

Miscellaneous

It is about time all these researchers, scientists, and the various diet kings get together and hash out their issues amongst one another. It is mind-blowing that there is so much miss-information regarding what we should eat, what we should avoid like the plague, and what we should consider cutting back on. This is where personal choice and no bullying come into play. Throughout this book, we have told you that you will not be bullied into choosing a lifestyle, and no one will force their opinions of what you should do. We are all able to make decisions, and you will make your decision based on what you feel is right for you.

Protein

Our bodies need protein to function. The essential amino acids that are found in protein are important to our overall well-being. Whether you want to believe it or not, protein helps build muscle mass, repairs damaged tissue, feeds cells, and produces hormones in your body. You can get your protein from many different sources such as animals, soy products, nuts, seeds, and legumes.

There is no need for you to give up on one lifestyle just to get the benefits of protein.

There are people who do not eat meat. It could be for a range of reasons such as disliking the taste or texture of animal-based products, or it could be for ethical or religious reasons. Whatever the reason or reasons, you have the freedom to make the decisions that are best for you.

Bone Broth

Homemade bone broth is full of nutritional goodness that will help in healing your gut lining, as well as protect your intestines from harmful bacteria. It also contains gelatin which helps by reducing inflammation and absorbing water to reinforce the stomach lining. Bone broth can be made from beef, chicken, or fish bones. You can purchase bone broth at the store, but homemade is better as you can control the additives. Bone broth is also an excellent base for many kinds of winter-warming soups.

Eggs

Whole eggs, that is egg white and yolk, are one of the healthiest foods you can get. They are jam-packed with all kinds of healthy vitamins, minerals, and nutrients to keep you, your eyes, and your brain working. Eggs are also filling, which will keep you full for longer periods between meals which will prevent snacking and assist with weight loss.

Fish

Let us take a moment here and imagine we are sitting at a seafood restaurant, overlooking the ocean and indulging in a mouthwatering fish taco, a pan-fried fillet of kingfish, or a perfectly grilled salmon. There is no way to sugarcoat this section, fish is the holy grail of health. Yes, fish is one of the healthiest types of food you can find.

There are thousands of different species and not all of them offer the same amount of nutrients, but your fishmonger at the market will be able to guide you if you want to know more. Known nutrients are vitamin D, omega-3 fatty acids, iodine, and minerals. The amount of goodness in fish is endless. Some of the benefits of including fish in your daily diet include improving your mood, reducing autoimmune diseases, improving eye health, and decreasing the chances of heart attacks and strokes.

Legumes

Legumes, love them or hate them, are high in protein, fiber, and vitamins which is beneficial for your army of bacteria. Some of the benefits of including legumes in your diet include reducing the bad cholesterol, stabilizing blood sugar levels, and growing your army of bacteria in healthy proportions. There are many legumes that can be eaten such as chickpeas, peas, beans, lentils, soybeans, and many more. Each of the variants offers different nutritional values such as the amount of protein it contains, the fiber content, and the various vitamins which are beneficial to your health and well-being.

Herbs and Spices

We have looked at all the different types of food we can eat that are beneficial in building up and strengthening our microbiome. You are probably assuming that the only way you can eat your food is by having no flavoring. We were saving the best for last. The condiments are the hidden treasures that add flavor to your meals, as well as added benefits such as keeping your army of critters happy and healthy.

Turmeric

Tumeric has become a popular spice over time. Not only is this Indian spice used in stews, curries, rice, and whatever else you think needs flavor, there are also medicinal properties. People have become creative in how they are using turmeric in their daily diet. Your army of microbiomes will be eternally grateful for the additional help as it helps with digesting your food, is an excellent anti-inflammatory, and features antibacterial properties to prevent stomach-related issues such as cramping and flatulence.

Cayenne Pepper

Your first thoughts when you see cayenne pepper are likely to compare it to chilies. Yes, that hot and burny little nugget that you can grow in your garden. You can use cayenne pepper to give your meals a kick and set your taste buds on fire, but did you know about the health benefits? Cayenne pepper has pretty much the same health properties which are boosting your metabolism, keeping you fuller for longer, helping with digestion, as well as sending healthy enzymes to your intestines.

Parsley

Parsley joins the ranks of either liking it or staying as far away from it as possible. It is commonly used in salads, soups, as a garnish, or in pasta dishes. Parsley is beneficial to the microbiome, in that it assists with digestion, acts as a diuretic and controls the emission of petrified gasses from your body. The general consensus is, that even if it takes an acquired set of taste buds to add it to your meals or smoothies, it will be the best move you can make for the overall health of your digestion.

Peppermint

This herb is not given enough credit amongst the community. Peppermint is associated with keeping your breath smelling good by sucking on a mint pastille, brushing your teeth, or using a minty mouthwash. Yes, this magic herb is very much underrated because it is so much more than the flavoring in our food and beauty care. Peppermint can be used to make tea by steeping a couple of leaves in hot water, which can be sipped after a hearty dinner to help with indigestion or alleviate stomach cramps. You can add the leaves to iced tea, infuse water, or garnish your salad with peppermint.

Miscellaneous

The most underrated part of any lifestyle has got to be the herbs and spices. Yes, we know and have known about their existence, but you probably never knew what the benefits were to your health. There are many herbs and spices we have not covered, which are beneficial to our microbiome and overall intestinal health. There are items we never got to list but are definitely worthwhile exploring at some stage such as cinnamon, cloves, fenugreek, ginger, and cardamon. The health benefits are plentiful ranging from regulating blood sugar levels, calming upset stomachs, and putting a damper on nausea to soothing inflamed intestines and preventing infections.

Chapter 8: Lifestyle Options And Sample Meal Plans

Lifestyle changes are a big deal to many. There are many reasons why a change in lifestyle is/was necessary. We understand how you are feeling, and we wanted to be with you on this journey. Until now, this has been an interesting trek as we have learned a lot. We have a better understanding of what is going on deep inside our bodies, in places that we took for granted. Having explored all the effects various foods have on our intestines has given us a greater respect for what we will eat or drink in the future.

Changes do not have to happen at once, we have learned that too. In order for any and all changes to be effective, we need to proceed at our own pace. We know where we are going wrong, and while we might deny some of these wrong-doings, we have been taking notes. Changes are imminent, as it is important to take care of ourselves. We are living in a world where things are changing with every second that goes by, and we understand the fear. There are those that say they are not afraid, but those that deny it the loudest are the ones that are more afraid. It is up to each and every one of us to be accountable for our health and well-being.

Do not be afraid to make changes. Remember who you are making the changes for. You want to improve your lifestyle and this is all about you. You are allowed to be selfish where your body is concerned. Start making changes today, whether you drink an extra glass of water or cut out one teaspoon of sugar, it is a start. You might have different reasons for wanting to change your lifestyle, whether it be for weight loss, overall wellness, or illnesses. Whatever the reason for your choice, ensure it is for the right reasons.

The time has come for us to have a look at a couple of the possible lifestyles you might like to adopt. Remember, there are hundreds of different types of diets for you to explore. If you have any pre-existing medical issues, please see your medical professional before making any changes to your diet or lifestyle. We want what is best for you, but only if your medical professional puts his/her stamp of approval on any changes you want to make. Your health and well-being are more important. It is important to remember that no diet or lifestyle change will have the same effect on everyone. What works for one, might not necessarily work for the other.

Every diet or lifestyle plan has a list of what they should be eating to either add fuel to their bodies, protect and nurture their intestines, or add beneficial nutrients. Similarly, there will also be a list of what you should eat less of and what you should not even think about looking at.

Again, no one is going to tell you that you must absolutely not eat this or that, but it is important to know the consequences it could create. Listen to your gut, it will be the first one to alert you when things are not working according to plan.

Mediterranean Diet

The first leg of our journey takes us to Italy and Greece. Well, technically we will be looking at how they incorporated the Mediterranean diet. This lifestyle transports us back in time when foods were not as processed as they are now. There have been studies that have proven that people who follow this lifestyle can ward off the risk of heart attacks, prevent strokes, and regulate blood sugar levels. As an added bonus, weight loss is a strong possibility.

Food List

Vegetables: broccoli, kale, cucumber, cauliflower, spinach, tomatoes, and carrots

Fruit: apples, oranges, strawberries, grapes, peaches, and pears

Root vegetables: potatoes, turnips, sweet potatoes, and yams

Whole grains: oats, brown rice, buckwheat, rye, and barley

Nuts: walnuts, macadamia, almonds, cashews, and hazelnuts

Legumes: lentils, chickpeas, beans, and peas

Seeds: pumpkin seeds, sunflower seeds, and flax seeds

Herbs: basil, thyme, sage, rosemary, cinnamon, and mint

Condiments: pepper, sea salt, and pink salt

Fish/seafood: salmon, tuna, mackerel, sardines, oysters, and mussels

Fats: extra virgin olive oil, avocados, olives, and avocado oil

Foods You Can Eat in Moderation

Poultry: chicken, quail, duck, and turkey

Eggs

Dairy: cheese, yogurt, and milk

Foods You Can Occasionally Eat

Red meat

Acceptable Beverages

Water

One glass of dry red wine

Herbal tea

Green tea

Chicory

Coffee

Kombucha

Foods and Beverages to Avoid

Added sugar such as soda, chocolates, and/or ice cream

Processed grains such as white bread and various pastas

Margarine

Refined oils such as canola oil and blended oils

Hot dogs, bologna, and basically everything that has been broken down and processed

Steer clear of anything that says low-fat, low-calories, or sugar-free. There are many more examples, but if it does not look natural, then it is not for you.

Fruit juices that have not been freshly made

Sample Meal Plan for the Mediterranean Diet

The following plan is to be used as a guide, and to indicate what a couple of days would look like when planning your way forward with the Mediterranean diet. You are free to make any changes by adding, removing, or switching anything that is not to your personal preference. You can be as creative as you like.

Day One

Breakfast: Unsweetened Greek yogurt, oats, and strawberries.

Lunch: A sandwich made from whole-grain bread, and a medley of vegetables.

Dinner: A tuna salad, with tomatoes, cucumber, and drizzled with olive oil - keep a helping for lunch on day two.

Dessert: A piece of fresh fruit.

Day Two

Breakfast: Oats and raisins.

Lunch: The leftover tuna salad.

Dinner: A Greek salad with tomatoes, feta cheese, and olives

Day Three

Breakfast: An omelet prepared with chopped up onion and tomatoes. Enjoy a fresh fruit as a treat.

Lunch: A sandwich made from whole-grain bread, packed with cheese and fresh vegetables.

Dinner: Homemade Mediterranean lasagne - portion some out for lunch on day four.

Day Four

Breakfast: Unsweetened yogurt with a selection of nuts and fresh fruit.

Lunch: Leftover lasagne.

Dinner: Broiled salmon on a bed of brown rice and a side of fresh vegetables.

Day Five

Breakfast: A stir fry of vegetables with eggs added, which are fried in olive oil.

Lunch: Unsweetened Greek yogurt with berries, nuts, and oats.

Dinner: A piece of grilled lamb, served with a nutritious salad, and a baked potato on the side.

Day Six

Breakfast: Oats with nuts and raisins, and an apple as a treat.

Lunch: A sandwich made from whole-grain bread, and a medley of fresh vegetables.

Dinner: A homemade Mediterranean pizza on a whole wheat base, packed with vegetables, olives, and a sprinkle of cheese - portion out a helping to enjoy for lunch on day seven.

Day Seven

Breakfast: An omelet with vegetables and olives.

Lunch: Leftover pizza.

Dinner: Grilled chicken, fresh vegetables, and a baked potato on the side.

Dessert: A choice of fresh fruit.

Healthy Snacks

If you find that you cannot survive on three meals a day, and you find yourself peckish between meals, opt for healthy treats instead of impulse-eating.

A handful of unflavored, raw nuts

Fresh fruit such as berries, grapes, or apples

Fresh vegetables such as carrots

Unsweetened Greek yogurt

Leftovers

The Mediterranean Diet in Summary

As lifestyles go, the Mediterranean diet seems to have eve-rything you would need to keep you interested and avoid be-ing bored. It does not appear to be restrictive, and you have the freedom to change the meal plan around to suit your day. It is easy to follow, no special foods are needed, and you can make do with what you have.

If you can follow the basic guidelines of this lifestyle, you will be able to reach whatever goals you have set for yourself. Whether your goal is to lose weight, eat correctly to correct any imbalances in your microbiome, or just that the time is right to take care of yourself, you will be able to achieve this without feeling deprived. The Mediterranean diet serves many purposes such as preventing and/or managing cardiovascular diseases and type 2 diabetes.

The Paleo Diet

Welcome to the next leg of our lifestyle-changing journey. Since the beginning of time, food has been a part of our lives. It is only fitting that we take a look at the paleo diet that has evolved from the time our cavemen ancestors realized they could eat. Way back then, the cavemen hunted for their food, ate natural foods - and probably dirt too, and lived to ripe old ages. Natural food back in the day was considered to be unprocessed and raw, which was beneficial to their lives.

As far as restricting diets go, the paleo diet is rather strict. The aim of this diet plan is to transport you back to the beginning of time and try to mimic the way our ancestors ate. The whole idea of the paleo diet is to limit the food that was introduced during the time when hunters and gatherers became farmers. According to loads of research and studies, the paleo diet is an ideal weight loss plan, as well as beneficial to the health and well-being of oneself.

Food List

Meat: pork, chicken, turkey, beef, and lamb

Seafood: trout, shellfish, salmon, and haddock

Eggs: high in omega 3, pastured, and free-range

Vegetables: peppers, onions, carrots, cauliflower, and kale

Fruits: tomatoes, berries, oranges, and apples

Root vegetables: yams, turnips, and potatoes

Unflavored nuts: cashews, macadamia, almonds, and walnuts

Raw seeds: flax, pumpkin, sunflower, and sesame

Healthy fats and oil: avocados, olives, extra virgin olive oils, and coconut oil

Condiments: sea salt, Himalayan salt, and pepper

Herbs: rosemary, sage, thyme, and turmeric

Dairy: full-fat milk, cheese, and butter

Food and Beverages to Avoid

Vegetable oils such as soybean, sunflower, and grapeseed

Anything with sugar such as ice cream, candy, soda, and fruit juice

Grains such as wheat, spelt, rye, and barley which are used to make pasta or bread

Legumes such as beans, peas, and lentils

Low-fat and fat-free dairy products

Margarine and anything that is labeled in the ingredients with the word "hydrogenated"

Ditch the artificial sweeteners that contain aspartame, sucralose, and saccharin

Diet, low-fat, and fat-free labeled foods are not recommended and should be avoided. Read the fine print on the packaging when in doubt and take note of all the additives and hidden "treasures" which are harmful to our bodies.

Sample Meal Plan for the Paleo Diet

The following meal plan is to be used as a guide for the paleo diet. You can amend the plan to make it suitable for your lifestyle and personal food preferences.

Day One

Breakfast: Fried eggs and vegetables prepared using coconut oil, and a piece of fresh fruit.

Lunch: A chicken salad with a drizzle of olive oil, and a handful of unflavoured nuts.

Dinner: A bunless burger fried in grass-fed butter, a side of vegetables, and homemade salsa. Portion out a helping for lunch the next day.

Day Two

Breakfast: Bacon and eggs, a piece of fresh fruit.

Lunch: The portioned leftover bunless burger, vegetables, and salsa.

Dinner: Salmon prepared in grass-fed butter, accompanied with a side of vegetables. Portion out a helping for the next day.

Day Three

Breakfast: Leftover salmon and vegetables.

Lunch: Time to get creative with a lettuce leaf sandwich or wrap filled with whatever permitted meat you have, topped with fresh vegetables.

Dinner: Grass-fed ground beef with vegetables. Portion out a helping for the next day.

Dessert: Berries as a sweet treat.

Day Four

Breakfast: Fried, scrambled, or boiled eggs, and a piece of fresh fruit.

Lunch: Leftover portion of ground beef and vegetables, and a handful of unflavored nuts.

Dinner: Pork fried in grass-fed butter or grilled, served with a side of vegetables.

Day Five

Breakfast: Fried eggs and vegetables prepared in coconut oil.

Lunch: A chicken salad with a drizzle of olive oil, and a handful of unflavoured nuts.

Dinner: Grilled steak served with a sweet potato and a side of salad. Portion out a helping for the next day.

Day Six

Breakfast: Bacon and eggs, with a piece of fresh fruit.

Lunch: Leftover grilled steak, and vegetables.

Dinner: Baked salmon with a side of vegetables, and an avocado salad. Portion out a helping for the next day.

Day Seven

Breakfast: Leftover salmon and vegetables from the night before.

Lunch: A lettuce leaf sandwich or wrap filled with whatever permitted meat you have, topped with fresh vegetables.

Dinner: Grilled chicken wings with a side of vegetables, and homemade salsa.

Healthy Snacks

If you find that you are feeling peckish between meals, opt for healthy treats instead of raiding the pantry.

Carrots

A piece of fresh fruit

A handful of unflavored nuts

Hard-boiled eggs

A bowl of fresh berries with coconut cream

Homemade beef jerky

The Paleo Diet in Summary

Following in the footsteps of our cavemen ancestors, the paleo diet takes us back in time before processed foods became a convenience and factories were used to modify our food. The paleo diet aims to take us back to the basics, where eating clean was considered a way of life. This lifestyle is easy to implement into your daily life. If following the basic guidelines by eliminating processed food from your daily intake, you will be on the road to a happy and healthier body.

The added bonus to adopting this diet is that it is adaptable to suit any lifestyle. It is easy to maintain without the feeling of being deprived. It is an affordable lifestyle, if you factor in the amount of money no longer used on processed, convenience, and junk food. If you want to get back to the basics and eat like your cavemen ancestors ate, give the paleo diet a try. Remember to consult your medical professional before implementing any changes.

Low-Carb Diet

This is going to be an interesting pit-stop on our journey. There is a lot of controversy surrounding the low-carb diet lifestyle. This has become a popular way of life, reaching the far corners of the world. Instead of choosing one of the popular names this lifestyle is associated with, we are using the simplest name to avoid being accused of favoritism. Some of the names that are associated with the low-carb diet are the ketogenic diet, the Atkins diet, and banting, to name a few.

The low-carb diet is rather restrictive in the food you may eat, even eliminating some food you would associate with being healthy. As with all the lifestyles we have looked at thus far, the low-carb diet will assist in shedding some unwanted pounds and amping up the energy levels as you become more comfortable with the changes.

Food List

Meat: beef, chicken, turkey, pork, and lamb

Fish: trout, kingfish, salmon, tuna, and haddock

Eggs: any eggs rich in omega 3, and pastured

Nuts: unflavored cashew, walnuts, and almonds

Seeds: sesame, flax, and pumpkin seeds

Vegetables: broccoli, cabbage, spinach, and cauliflower

Fruits: berries, apples, and pears

Dairy: hard cheese, full fat and Greek yogurt, and cream

Fats: grass-fed butter, coconut oil, olive oil, and lard

Legumes: lentils, pinto beans, and peas

Beverages: unsweetened tea and coffee, and water

Food and Beverages to Avoid

Sugar is found in sodas, fruit juice, ice-cream, and candy. In other words, anything that has sugar in it should be sent to a sugary grave.

Wheat, rice, barley, bread, cereal, and pasta.

Margarine and anything that is labeled in the ingredients with the word "hydrogenated".

Any and all products with the labels "low fat" and "diet" should be eliminated from your pantry, fridge, and home.

Certain vegetables that are higher in carbohydrate content than normal vegetables, also known as starchy vegetables.

Sample Menu Plan for the Low-Carb Diet

Day One

Breakfast: An omelet with vegetables, and prepared using coconut oil or butter.

Lunch: Unsweetened yogurt with berries and almonds.

Dinner: A bunless burger, topped with cheese, a side of vegetables and a homemade salsa sauce. Portion out a helping for the next day.

Day Two

Breakfast: Bacon and eggs fried in lard.

Lunch: Leftover cheeseburger, vegetables, and salsa.

Dinner: Pan-fried salmon in butter, with a side of vegetables.

Day Three

Breakfast: Fried or scrambled eggs prepared in coconut oil or butter, and vegetables.

Lunch: A hearty shrimp salad served with salad greens and drizzled with olive oil.

Dinner: Grilled chicken served with a side of vegetables.

Day Four

Breakfast: An omelet and vegetables prepared with coconut oil or butter.

Lunch: A berry smoothie with almonds and coconut milk.

Dinner: Grilled steak and a serving of vegetables.

Day Five

Breakfast: Bacon and eggs prepared with lard.

Lunch: A hearty grilled chicken salad with a drizzle of olive oil.

Dinner: Grilled pork chop with a healthy serving of vegetables.

Day Six

Breakfast: An omelet prepared with butter or coconut oil, and filled with vegetables.

Lunch: Unsweetened yogurt with berries, coconut flakes,

and some unflavored nuts.

Dinner: Meatballs served on a bed of vegetables.

Day Seven

Breakfast: Bacon and eggs prepared with lard.

Lunch: A chocolate and berry smoothie with cocoa powder, heavy cream, and coconut milk.

Dinner: Grilled chicken wings served on a bed of raw spinach, and dressed with an olive oil dressing.

Healthy Snacks

If you are eating enough vegetables, protein and fats, you should be sated. If, for some reason, your brain is convincing you that you are about to keel over from hunger, consider eating the following snacks to satisfy you.

A full-fat unsweetened yogurt

A hard-boiled egg

Any leftovers you might have

Hard cheese

Berries

Unflavoured nuts

The Low-Carb Diet in Summary

In a nutshell, this is an interesting lifestyle change. As already mentioned, it is rather restrictive but it is doable. In order for you to feel like this could work for you, you will have to pull those sugar and snack-craving teeth.

You are stronger than you think you are. If you want the changes hard enough, you absolutely, most definitely, will succeed.

The Vegan Lifestyle

We could not list all these meaty lifestyles without thinking of our plant-based lifestyle friends! Again, if we had to leave out the vegetarians and vegans, we would be in a whole lot of trouble and blamed for being meat lovers. In fact, that is far from the truth, as all the plans thus far can be tweaked and manipulated to exclude any animal by-products.

We are all aware of the jokes surrounding the plant-based lifestyles, and this is a lifestyle adopted by people who decided not to eat anything animal-related. This is a huge change for a meat-lover but also a satisfying outcome if you were struggling with some health issues such as cholesterol or high blood pressure. A complete change in lifestyle can impact your health in more than one positive way, and a big change is losing weight. Yes, whatever you think about a plant-based diet, you might change your views and join the millions who have already embarked on this new lifestyle.

There are a lot of people who do not understand, or maybe they do not want to understand, the concept of eliminating all animal-produced protein and products. It is not up to us to judge anyone for their chosen lifestyles.

There could be many reasons for the decision such as ethical, religious, environmental, or health reasons. The health benefits of a plant-based lifestyle far outweigh any negative comments from people who find it necessary to criticize. The plant-based lifestyle helps with keeping the heart happy, controlling blood sugar levels, and preventing chronic diseases.

Shopping List

Instead of giving a food list, we will be giving you a shopping list of what you might need if you want to follow this lifestyle. This is only a guide of what your options would look like.

Fresh is Best

Vegetables: cabbage, carrots, cauliflower, potatoes, eggplant, zucchini, and many more

Fruit: berries, cherries, citrus, kiwis, pomegranates, and many more

Grains

Brown rice

Lentils

Buckwheat

Oats

Quinoa

Carbohydrates

Whole wheat pasta

Brown rice wraps

Wild rice

Plant-Based Protein

Unflavored nuts: Brazil, cashews, peanuts, pistachio, pecans, and many more

Seeds: chia, flax, hemp, pumpkin, sesame, sunflower, and many more

Legumes: chickpeas, black beans, lentils, pinto beans, kidney beans, and many more

Soy: tempeh, tofu, edamame, and many more

Dairy

Milk: almond, coconut, oat, rice, cashew, and soy milks

Cheese: vegan parmesan

Egg Substitute

Cornstarch

Arrowroot powder

Aquafaba

Silken tofu

Fats

Avocado oil

Olive oil

Tahini

Flaxseed oil

Coconut oil

Snacks

Dark chocolate

Hummus

Nut butters

Popcorn

Roasted chickpeas

Seaweed crisps

Sweeteners

Coconut sugar

Dates

Stevia

Molasses

Spices

Cinnamon

Garlic powder

Cumin

Chili powder

Turmeric

Pepper

Herbs

Thyme

Rosemary

Sage

Paprika

Basil

Sample Menu Plan for the Vegan Lifestyle

Day One

Breakfast: Tempeh bacon served with mushrooms, on a bed of wilted arugula, and a side of avocado.

Lunch: Vegan meatballs made with lentils, whole wheat pasta, and a side of salad,

Dinner: Cauliflower and chickpea tacos, topped with guacamole.

Day Two

Breakfast: Coconut yogurt with chia seeds, unflavoured nuts, and berries.

Lunch: Tofu on a bed of herb-flavored couscous, with a side of sauteed cabbage, and Brussel sprouts.

Dinner: A mushroom lentil loaf, with a side of green beans, and cauliflower.

Day Three

Breakfast: Peanut butter and banana on sweet potato toast.

Lunch: A tempeh taco filled with quinoa, onions, beans, cilantro, tomatoes, and topped with avocado.

Dinner: Swiss chard, mushrooms, and butternut, served on oat risotto.

Day Four

Breakfast: Quiche with broccoli, tomatoes, spinach, and silken tofu.

Lunch: Spinach and chickpea curry, served on brown rice.

Dinner: A lentil salad with Mediterranean vegetables such as peppers, cucumbers, sun-dried tomatoes, olives, and kale.

Day Five

Breakfast: Oats soaked overnight and topped with an apple slice, pumpkin seeds, cinnamon, and nut butter.

Lunch: Black bean burger, served with a side of vegetables and sweet potato wedges.

Dinner: Vegan mac and cheese, with a side of collard greens.

Day Six

Breakfast: Tempeh, broccoli, kale, zucchini, and tomatoes.

Lunch: Tofu stir-fried with vegetables and quinoa, and seasoned with garlic and ginger.

Dinner: Black-eyed peas bean salad with corn, peppers, onions, and tomatoes.

Day Seven

Breakfast: Whole-grain toast topped with avocado, and washed down with a protein shake.

Lunch: Lentil chili, a baked potato, and a side of grilled asparagus.

Dinner: A medley of vegetables featuring onion, peppers, artichoke, tomatoes, and chickpeas, served on brown rice.

The Vegan Lifestyle in Summary

This has truly been an inspirational section of this book. Whether you agree with the vegan lifestyle or not, it should not be dismissed by anyone. For a start, all the food mentioned throughout this section is all microbiome-friendly. You can literally feel your intestines doing a happy jiggle at reading the different food types. Yes, we know that die-hard meat lovers will stick you in a hole if you decide to convert, but ask yourself if they are the type of people you want to be acquainted with? People that would judge you for wanting to try something new, as well as giving yourself a body, mind, and health makeover. Do what is right for you. Be selfish, and think only of yourself. No, absolutely no judgment here.

The Microbiome Diet

This is the final stop on our journey to explore various lifestyles. As far as lifestyles and diets go, we will be closing the door after this one. The microbiome diet is a plan that was put together by Dr. Raphael Kellman, who specializes in the microbiome and how our intestines work. We will not be rehashing what the microbiome is and what it does for us, as that would be a whole lot of repeating. Refresh your memory from the prior chapters if necessary.

The microbiome diet is a three-phase program. Each phase will take you closer to the end goal, which is resetting your microbiome and retraining your microbiome to work with the new and improved bacteria and enzymes. The first phase will be removing the evil bacteria and dispersing the prebiotics and probiotics to begin the all-important healing process in the gut lining. Are you ready to get started?

Phase One

The first phase is said to be the hardest of the three phases. It will last 21 days, and it will take a lot of determination and perseverance to reach the end.

After the ensuing 21 days, you will have retrained your gut. By following the guide, you will have flushed the unhealthy critters from your gut, and built up your stomach acids and digestive enzymes to help churn the food so that magic and healing can happen on the inside. We will achieve the desired outcome by implementing and sticking to the first phase of this new lifestyle which is known as the "Four R's Meal Plan", for 21 days.

Remove

Before you make any radical changes to your lifestyle or eating plan, speak to your medical professional. If you are taking prescription medication for chronic conditions, do not just stop taking them without consulting with a professional. The idea in this part of phase one is to eliminate all food, harmful chemicals, and toxins that would or could cause inflammation and disrupt your army of healthy critters.

Repair

Visit the local farmer's market and stock up on prebiotic- and probiotic-rich vegetables.

These include asparagus, garlic, leeks, onions, and Jerusalem artichokes. Stock up on fermented foods, or even better, start learning how to make your own. There will be a recipe on this process in the next chapter, so you will be able to save money, as well as make your very own probiotic produce such as sauerkraut and kimchi.

Replace

Instead of relying on the store-bought spices which are high in sugar and salt, opt for natural herbs and spices which are beneficial to your health. These herbs and spices have an holistic advantage that can replace the acid in your stomach, fine-tune your digestive system, and help you feel good in the depths of your gut. These herbs and spices include Tumeric, cloves, cinnamon, and dandelion.

Reinoculate

Do not be shy about filling your gut with healthy bacteria and feeding those bacteria with their special food that will help them grow stronger the more they are nourished.

As you can see, phase one is rather strict and regimented. It is all part of the greater scheme of the plan, which is to take care of the part of the body that is often neglected and abused the most, the stomach. During phase one, you will be eliminating all grains, dairy, eggs, and fruit and vegetables which are high in starch. You will also want to avoid fried foods, fast foods, sugar, artificial sweeteners, and basically everything that has been processed to the hilt. The focus is on all the healthy, prebiotic- and probiotic-rich foods which are going to be repairing a lot of damage. Supplements such as zinc, vitamin D, grapefruit seed extract, and oregano oil are recommended. See you in 21 days for the second phase.

Phase Two

Welcome back! Phase one lasted forever. You were probably ready to give up on day one, but you stuck it out and persevered for 21 days. You are ready to move on to the second stepping stone. Before we move on to the next 28 days of your gut rejuvenation reclamation, we want to assure you that the 21 days were not designed to torture you. As we have mentioned repeatedly throughout this book, you are not being forced to do anything you do not want to do. We also assured you that these are not diets, even though they may mimic the diets we have all come to hate, these are lifestyle changes.

Over the last 21 days of phase one, you have retrained your brain to think about food differently. You are ingesting food you probably would not have looked at, let alone tasted, a month or two ago. You made the decision to change, no one forced you. Keeping in mind the changes you went through during phase one, phase two might be a little easier as you are being introduced to a variety of food. We should actually say that you are being reintroduced to food.

By day one of 28, we are hopeful that your microbiome has gotten stronger and that you feel energized. As we start on the second phase of this lifestyle, you are going to start adding some food that was restricted during phase one. Do not go and eat everything you can lay your hands on, that will just be defeating all the hard work you have already achieved. You can start adding dairy, eggs, legumes, and gluten-free grains into your daily intake. In addition, you can also start eating some of the forbidden fruit and vegetables such as peaches, pears, and sweet potatoes. We look forward to seeing you in 28 days.

Phase Three

Welcome back to the third phase of the microbiome diet. How are you feeling? The good news is, you have reached the end of the counting days. All that is left now is the maintenance phase. Yes, phase three is maintaining what you have accomplished over the last 49 days. However, you should remain in this phase until you have reached and maintained whatever goals you set out to start with. The recommendation is that you continue avoiding the foods you were cautioned to cut out and abandon in phase one, as you have done an amazing job of healing your microbiome. In addition to the healing, you have learned how to get along without the temptations that could have potentially caused you to have a heart attack, a stroke, or develop diabetes.

All that matters now is that you did something magnificent for yourself. You put your health first, and that should be something you could celebrate by having an extra helping of sauerkraut. Okay, we said we wouldn't use food as a reward system, so possibly a visit to the hair salon or a relaxing massage is called for.

Sample Meal Plan for the Microbiome Diet

The following plan is to be used as a guide. This is a three-day plan from phase one.

Day One

Breakfast: A fresh fruit salad, and unflavored Brazil nuts.

Mid-morning snack: Parsnip sticks prepared with almond butter.

Lunch: A chicken and fresh vegetable soup.

Mid-afternoon snack: Curry-roasted cauliflower.

Dinner: Roasted Brussel sprouts, a mixed greens salad, fermented beets, and a perfectly grilled fillet of salmon.

Day Two

Breakfast: Almond flour pancakes with fresh fruit and almond butter.

Mid-morning snack: Nuts and berries.

Lunch: A hearty vegetable salad featuring chickpeas and sauerkraut, splashed with a parsley-lemon vinaigrette.

Mid-afternoon snack: Homemade guacamole and celery sticks.

Dinner: Chicken meatballs soaking in a marinara sauce on a bed of zucchini noodles.

Day Three

Breakfast: Breakfast cookies made with almond flour and blueberries.

Mid-morning snack: Pan-fried pineapple with crunchy coconut.

Lunch: Miso-glazed cod served with a healthy serving of vegetable salad.

Mid-afternoon snack: Hummus and carrot sticks.

Dinner: Steak tacos served with steamed vegetables, guacamole, and salsa.

Food List

River salmon

Grass-fed meats

Fermented vegetables such as sauerkraut, beets, kimchi, and carrots

Prebiotic-rich vegetables such as asparagus, garlic, leeks, onions, and artichokes

Fruits such as apples, cherries, grapefruit, oranges, nectarines, and tomatoes

Unflavoured nuts

Seeds

Nut butters

Herbs such as basil, rosemary, peppermint, and sage

Spices such as turmeric, cinnamon, and cayenne pepper

In Summary

As with all lifestyle changes, whether it be cutting out this or that or adopting a new way of life, there will be the urge to resist the changes. You will experience cravings you never thought possible. Your brain is telling you that if you don't eat that piece of candy, the world is going to explode. News flash, the world exploded the day a virus started spreading faster than a wildfire in a small area. You will survive these intense cravings. Keep yourself busy by practicing a new hobby, dancing, meditating, or cleaning your house from top to bottom. Be strong and be positive. Stare ahead and imagine the winners ribbon at the end of a marathon. Now envision a crowd of smiling cells, bacteria, fungi, and viruses with their pom-poms. They are cheering you on because you overcame the challenges. They are happy because they have been rejuvenated. You are happy because you feel better than you have ever felt.

Remember who you are making the changes for. Keep that end goal in your vision at all times.

At the end of the day, the different lifestyles we have presented to you are only an outline of what is available to you. There are thousands of variations of the same lifestyles/diets, and there are many other types of diets out there. The low-carb diet might be wonderful for Jonah, but it might have the opposite effect on Jocelyn. Some people need more carbs in their diets, where other people cannot look at a slice of bread or a potato without feeling bloated or gaining 10 pounds by glancing at it. Before starting or thinking about starting a new diet, inspect the food lists of what is allowed and what is not allowed. Make your notes. Write down your questions. Visit your doctor, discuss your intentions on which lifestyle you would like to adopt, and see if the option you have chosen is the right one. Remember, your doctor or medical professional will want what is best for you.

Sugar addiction is real. As are the cravings for salty and fried foods. It is an ongoing struggle but if you are determined to make the best of the positive changes you want to implement in your lifestyle, you will learn how to overcome this battle. It is like smoking, you have to take it one day at a time in order to be successful. Do not plan ahead of time by telling everyone that you will not be eating sugar for the week. That will be at the forefront of every thought you have, and you will have your brain convincing you that it needs sugar or you need that cookie. Take each moment as it comes.

Chapter 9: Recipes

After a very long journey, where we discovered things we might have known but never really understood, or known but never thought about, we have reached the part of the book where you can venture to be creative with the food you eat. We have looked at a couple of different lifestyles you can adopt, or you can have the freedom to find a lifestyle that will suit you.

We are now going to share some recipes which can be adapted to suit what is permitted on your lifestyle plan. Be creative. Do not limit yourself. Recipes are guides and you can play with them by adding your own unique flair. At the end of the day, you are the one that is going to be eating the food, and we do not want you to feel as if you have been forced to eat food you do not like. We want you to be happy with your choices.

Breakfast

Spinach and Feta Breakfast Wrap

Spinach, feta, and olives are a match made in heaven. Your breakfast wrap can be made on the go, or you can pre-make them and freeze them for the days when you are pressed for time. You can add onions, peppers, chopped chicken, chilies, or whatever your taste buds feel like exploring. You can make your scrambled egg using only egg whites for the extra protein kick. If you want a vegan breakfast, exchange the eggs for a vegan egg substitute or silken tofu, and use vegan cheese instead of feta.

Time: 10 minutes

Serving Size: 1 wrap

Prep Time: 5 minutes

Cook Time: 5 minutes

Ingredients:

- 2 eggs

- ½ cup of chopped spinach

- 4 olives which have been chopped

- ¼ cup of crumbled feta cheese

- 1 ½ tablespoons of grass-fed butter - cubed

- Salt and pepper taste

- 1 white or whole wheat tortilla wrap

Directions:

1. Gather all your ingredients before you start cooking.

2. Whisk the eggs in a separate bowl.

3. Melt ½ tablespoon of butter over medium heat in a small frying pan. Swirl the pan to ensure it is coated with the butter.

4. Add the rest of the cubed butter to the egg mixture, and season with salt and pepper.

5. Add the egg mixture to the heated pan.

6. Allow eggs to rest for a minute or two.

7. Using a spatula, gently move the egg around until nearly cooked.

8. Add spinach and mix together until cooked.

9. Spoon the egg and spinach mixture on the tortilla, and add feta cheese and olives.

10. Wrap and enjoy.

Caprese Avocado Toast

A hearty open-toasted sandwich topped with nothing but goodness. You can never go wrong with a combination of avocado, fresh tomatoes, basil, cheese or the sweet tangy taste of balsamic glaze. A nourishing breakfast that can be enjoyed for lunch, snack time, or dinner.

Time: 7 minutes

Serving Size: 2

Prep Time: 5 minutes

Cook Time: 2 minutes

Ingredients:

- 2 slices of wholesome bread such as sourdough, whole wheat, or peasant bread

- 1 medium avocado which has been halved and pitted

- 8 grape tomatoes cut in halves

- 2 ounces of bite-sized mozzarella balls

- 4 large basil leaves shredded

- 2 tablespoons of balsamic glaze

Directions:

1. Put the bread in the toaster or a toaster oven.

2. While bread is toasting, mash avocado.

3. Add avocado liberally over the toast.

4. Add tomatoes, mozzarella, and shredded basil.

5. Add a drizzle of balsamic glaze.

6. Serve immediately and enjoy.

Lunch

Pan-Seared Citrus Shrimp Recipe (Part One)

This delicious salad can be enjoyed for lunch, or as a re-freshing dinner on a hot summer's night. It is just the right blend of everything that is healthy and packed with essential nutrients. This is a two-part recipe, as we will have to cook the shrimp first and assemble the salad in part two. Let's get shrimping.

Time: 15 minutes

Serving Size: 6

Prep Time: 5 minutes

Cook Time: 10 minutes

Ingredients:

- 1 tablespoon olive oil

- 1 cup of freshly squeezed orange juice

- ½ a cup of freshly squeezed lemon juice

- 5 garlic cloves either pressed or minced

- 1 tablespoon of red onion, or shallot which has been finely chopped

- 1 tablespoon of finely chopped fresh parsley

- 3 pounds of medium shrimp which have been deveined, peeled and cleaned

- 1 medium orange cut into wedges

- 1 medium lemon cut into wedges

- A pinch of red pepper flakes

- Kosher salt and fresh ground black pepper to taste

Directions:

Whisk together olive oil, orange and lemon juice, garlic, onion, 2 teaspoons of parsley, and red pepper flakes.

1. Pour the mixture into a large skillet over medium heat.

2. Allow to simmer and cook the mixture for about five to eight minutes, until it has been reduced by half.

3. Add the shrimp, and season to taste.

4. Cover and allow shrimp to simmer in the reduction until they turn pink.

5. Sprinkle remaining parsley over the cooked shrimp, and serve with lemon and orange wedges on the side.

Citrus Shrimp Salad with Avocado (Part Two)

Time: 5 minutes

Serving Size: 4

Prep Time: 5 minutes

Cook Time: N/A

Ingredients:

- 1 pound of the pan-seared citrus shrimp

- 8 cups of greens (arugula, spinach, or lettuce)

- 1 avocado, pitted and sliced

- 1 shallot, minced

- 4 ounces of toasted, sliced almonds

- Lemon- or fruit-flavored extra virgin olive oil

- Lemon or orange juice

- Kosher salt and freshly ground black pepper to taste

Directions:

1. Add the greens to a large salad bowl.

2. Toss a helping of shrimp in with the greens, either warm or cold.

3. Drizzle with olive oil.

4. Leftover sauce from the cooking process can be added if desired.

5. Toss the greens and shrimp to coat with oil and/or sauce.

6. Add sliced avocado, shallots, and almonds.

7. Season with salt and pepper to taste.

8. Serve and enjoy.

Dinner

Whole30 Chicken Meatballs and Cauliflower Rice with Coconut-Herb Sauce

There is no need to deprive yourself of your favorite comfort foods. With some tweaks and adjustments, you can eat anything you want. This recipe can be tweaked by using ground beef or ground turkey. The meatballs can be made in bulk, portioned out, and frozen. You can add or remove any herbs and spices to suit your palate.

Time: 45 minutes

Serving Size: 4 servings

Prep Time: 25 minutes

Cook Time: 20 minutes

Ingredients for the Meatballs:

- 1 tbsp extra virgin olive oil
- ½ a red onion
- 2 garlic cloves minced
- 1 lb ground chicken
- ¼ cup of chopped parsley
- 1 tbsp of Dijon mustard
- ¾ tsp kosher salt
- ½ tsp freshly ground black pepper
- Nonstick spray

Ingredients for the Sauce:

- One 14-ounce can coconut milk
- 1 ¼ cups fresh parsley chopped and divided
- 4 scallions chopped
- 1 garlic clove which has been peeled and crushed
- The juice and zest of one lemon
- Kosher salt and freshly ground black pepper

- Red pepper flakes

Directions for the Meatballs:

1. Start off by turning on the oven to 375°F.

2. Line your baking sheet with aluminum foil.

3. Liberally spray with nonstick spray.

4. Heat your olive oil over a medium heat in a skillet pan.

5. Add the onion to the warm pan and saute for about five minutes.

6. Add the garlic, and let the garlic and the onion fuse together for a minute.

7. Remove the onion and garlic mixture from the heat, and allow to cool.

8. Season the ground chicken by adding the parsley, mustard, salt, and pepper.

9. Add the onion and garlic mixture to the seasoned ground chicken.

10. Roll the mixture into any size balls you require, small, medium, or large.

11. Place the rolled meatballs on the prepared baking sheet.

12. Bake until fully cooked and feeling firm, roughly between 17 to 20 minutes.

13. Sprinkle with red pepper flakes and parsley.

Directions for the Sauce:

1. Place the coconut milk, parsley, garlic, lemon zest, lemon juice, and scallions into the food processor.

2. Blitz the ingredients together until well blended.

3. Add the salt and pepper.

4. Pour a generous helping of sauce over your meatballs and serve on a bed of cauliflower rice.

Cauliflower Rice

Cauliflower rice has become increasingly popular in households where people are following low-carb lifestyles. As the recipe above calls for cauliflower rice, we have decided to add it to this chapter. It can be used in any meal, or it can be used to bind foods together. Cauliflower rice can be used for all kinds of experiments, and whatever you decide on, Jamie Oliver will be proud of you.

Time: 20 minutes

Serving Size: 6 servings

Prep Time: 15 minutes

Cook Time: 5 minutes

Ingredients:

- 1 head of cauliflower

- A splash of olive oil

- Freshly ground black pepper and sea salt to taste

Directions:

1. Break the head of cauliflower apart, into florets.

2. Rinse the florets and pat dry.

3. Pulse the cauliflower in a food processor until it looks like refined rice.

4. Continue until all the cauliflower has been processed.

5. The cauliflower rice is ready to eat raw, or you can cook it by sauteing till the desired tenderness is reached.

6. For a cold dish, you can drizzle in some olive oil and season with salt and pepper.

7. For a warm dish, you can fry the cauliflower rice in olive oil for two to three minutes, season with salt and pepper, and top it with meatballs and sauce, roasted vegetables, and just about anything that is delicious.

Dessert/Snacks

Healthy Peanut Butter Pie

No matter what lifestyle or diet you are following, guilt-free desserts and snacks are mandatory. If anyone wants to argue this point, they will have to be ready for an epic battle. In all seriousness, a guilt-free treat is always welcome.

Time: 3 hours and 25 minutes

Serving Size: 10 slices

Prep Time: 25 minutes

Cook Time: 3 hours

Ingredients for the Pie Crust:

- 1 cup of unflavored walnuts or pecan nuts

- 1 cup of unflavored cashews

- 2 tbsp honey or maple syrup

- 2 to 4 tbsp of milk - coconut, almond, cow or soy milk

- 2 tsp vanilla extract

- 1 tsp cinnamon

- ¼ tsp salt

Ingredients for the Peanut Butter Filling

- 1 cup of unsweetened and unsalted plain peanut butter

- 3 ripe bananas, medium-sized

- 3 tbsp of milk - coconut, almond, cow or soy milk

- 2 tsp vanilla extract

- ¼ tsp salt

- ⅓ cup of dark chocolate chips

Directions for the Pie Crust:

1. Add 1 cup of walnuts, 1 cup of cashews, 2 tbsp of honey, 2 tbsp of milk, 2 tsp of vanilla extract, 1 tsp of cinnamon, and ¼ tsp of salt in the food processor.

2. Mix together until everything is blended together.

3. Add some milk, and continue adding until the desired consistency is reached.

4. Take care not to over-process your crust.

5. Turn the dough into a 9-inch pie dish.

6. Press the dough into the pie dish to cover the base and sides.

Directions for the Peanut Butter Filling

1. Add 1 cup of peanut butter, 3 ripe bananas, 3 tbsp of milk, 2 tsp vanilla extract, and ¼ salt to the food processor.

2. Blend until smooth.

3. Pour the peanut butter filling into the pie shell and smooth.

4. Top with chocolate chips.

5. Cover with saran wrap and pop in the freezer until frozen.

6. When you are ready for your sweet treat, thaw before enjoying a slice.

Frozen Yogurt Covered Blueberries

A lifestyle change does not mean the end of the world. Yes, you made some healthy changes and ditched the sugar. That is no reason to completely give up on your snacks. Enjoy this delicious, guilt-free treat. This nutritious snack is the ideal treat to enjoy on a hot summer's night.

Time: 1 hour and 10 minutes

Serving Size: 2 servings

Prep Time: 10 minutes

Cook Time: 1 hour

Ingredients:

- 6 oz of fresh blueberries

- 6 oz of blueberry Greek yogurt

- Optional extras include honey, vanilla, or strawberry

Directions:

1. Wash the blueberries and pat dry.

2. Line a baking sheet with wax paper.

3. By using a toothpick, dip a blueberry in the yogurt, ensuring the blueberry is coated.

4. Place onto the baking sheet.

5. Continue with steps 2 and 4 until all the berries are coated.

6. Place the baking sheet in the freezer for at least an hour, or until the berries have frozen.

7. You can put the frozen blueberries in a container and keep it in the freezer. Then enjoy a guilt-free snack any time you have a craving.

Fermentation Guide

The recipe you have been waiting for, the basic guide to fermenting your own produce. As you know, fermented vegetables are an excellent source of probiotics.

Time: 4 to 10 days

Serving Size: 8 - 10 servings

Prep Time: 4 to 10 days

Ingredients:

- Your choice of vegetables, sliced, diced, or chopped
- Wash vegetables thoroughly, and pat dry
- 2 cups of water
- 1 ½ tbsp of coarse sea salt
- 1 cabbage leaf
- Your choice of herbs and spices
- Wide-mouth mason jars
- Plastic lids

Directions:

1. Fill the mason jars with vegetables, herbs, and spices.

2. Leave a gap of at least an inch from the top of the jar.

3. Mix the salt and water together until no salt crystals remain.

4. Add the saltwater over the vegetables, leaving ½ an inch of space from the top.

5. Add a folded cabbage leaf and place it over the vegetables, making sure that the cabbage leaf keeps the vegetables covered by the saltwater. ****This is not necessary and can be skipped if desired.****

6. Secure the lid as tight as possible.

7. Avoid sunlight and place it where the temperature is between 68 to 75 degrees Fahrenheit.

8. When you notice bubbling after a few days, gently open the lid to allow the gas out. You can repeat this process one or two times a day.

9. Your vegetables will be ready from day four onwards.

10. The longer you leave them to ferment, the more they mature.

11. The taste testing can commence from day four until you have reached your desired preference.

12. When you have reached your preference, you can store your jars in the refrigerator.

13. All that is left is to enjoy your very own, homemade fermented vegetables. Your microbiome will be forever indebted to you.

Conclusion

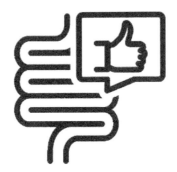

We have reached the part of the book where you are either elated that it is ending, or that you would like to continue. This journey has opened our eyes and given us an insight into what is going on inside us. Whether we like to admit it or not, we are deeply regretting all the trauma we have inflicted on our bodies. We are equipped with some knowledge on how we are able to repair the damage and how to implement some necessary changes.

At the beginning of this journey, we couldn't stress enough that this is not about forcing you into a corner and making you do something you do not want to do. What we presented you with was a couple of lifestyles you could use to make changes. This book is and was not intended for any specific body type. Whether you weigh 100 pounds or 230 pounds, the aim of this book was to take a microscopic look into your body and identify possible causes of any illnesses, diseases, general health concerns.

We hope you have an understanding of what is going on in the chambers of your body which you've always known exists but never fully understood the functions. If you never knew what the microbiome was before you started reading this book, you were probably slightly grossed out when you began to realize that your body is home to trillions of viruses, fungi, and bacteria that actually keep us healthy. Now you can giggle at your initial response upon finding out and appreciate the impact these little bugs have on your health and well-being.

Our Promise

At the very beginning, during, and at every opportunity we could, we promised and assured you that no one would be forcing you into choosing a new lifestyle. What we did was present you with a couple of options that could be altered to suit your personal preferences. Everyone is quick to offer advice, which is actually judgment from where we are on the outside looking in, about what you should eat or not eat to shed some stubborn pounds. Our lifestyle suggestions could lead to you losing a pound or three, but that is not the intention. The intention was that we would not judge each other for the decisions we made in the past or will make in the future. We were intent on correcting what was wrong, so that we can be around a little longer to torment those judge Judy's.

Remember, even when you have read the last word in this chapter, it does not mean that this is the end. We will be around for you whenever you want a refresher or some encouragement when you are feeling despondent. You will never be alone on this journey. You are going to eat your way to a new and improved microbiome, and you are going to testify to the masses how easy it is to change the way we see food.

Food for Thought

Food is not the enemy, so do not be afraid to enjoy your meals. Food has no power over you, you have the power. We gave you a couple of recipes that are versatile and can be adjusted to include or exclude anything according to your preferences. There are even two mouth-watering snack/dessert ideas which you can indulge in without the guilt! Who would have thought that you could create guilt-free treats while filling your body with nutrients to ward off infections and diseases? Be as creative as you want to be, even if the flavor combinations make no sense to anyone else.

Be Kind to Yourself

Do not be so hard on yourself. Do not let your past define your future. You are starting a new chapter in your life, one where you have made the decision to change your ways. You will stumble and fall along the way. You will indulge in a triple cheeseburger with fries drenched in ranch dressing. You will go to a party, or an evening out with friends, and have a few too many drinks. You are allowed to live. You are allowed to break free from the chains. We have said this over and over again, everything in moderation. Please do not see you breaking out as a sign of weakness and that all hope is lost. Tomorrow is another day, where you can start over. Your gut microbiome is more forgiving than you give it credit for. Embrace your new lifestyle journey.

It Is Time...

It is time to turn you loose and to let you decide on your next steps going forward. Thank you for joining us on this eye-opening, gut-revealing journey of discovery, where you have discovered how you can take control of your health.

If you would like to continue on, don't forget to subscribe to the newsletter for your free short article: some personal thoughts on other implications of the microbiome functions: https://tinyurl.com/jsalutelli. You'll also receive the update on our new publications.

Reviews help authors more than you might think, especially for a first-time writer. If you enjoyed *Friendly Microbiome*, please consider leaving a review on your online bookstore—it would be greatly appreciated.

We hope you enjoyed your time learning with us. It definitely was a journey that taught us to appreciate the food we eat and opened the door for us to explore new food. We hope you learned how to be kind to yourself and how not to knock yourself down. Be true to who you are!

About The Author

Throughout my last five years working and living abroad in an Asian country, I realized I was overwhelmed by my frenetic life, job tasks, customer visits, married life and general pressures. All this led me to forget about my health, leaving no time to exercise (that was the excuse I was telling myself...), and, most important, neglecting my diet and quality of life. Soon, I started to gain weight, and no matter how much I tried to go back to gym and work out, I was still unsatisfied by my body and the feelings I had. My problems were partially due to my low-quality lifestyle and pressure covering my entire week, but most of all, they were caused by my bad habits and the food and beverages I was consuming.

I started a personal path that brought me back to what I studied about nutrition and medicine, and I expanded my knowledge about the wellness and the peace of mind and body. I got back on track, imposing limits to my professional life and dedicating more time to myself and my family. I realized I could have all the time I needed to follow my hobbies and really enjoy my free time. I improved my sleep quality, which had a variety of positive results. I started to lose weight without exhausting diets and rigid programs; I just had to change my nutrition base concepts, avoid bad habits and focus on gut friendly foods and my circadian rhythm.

The results I had, which can help to have a longer life, are not hard to reach. What I need at the time was to first change my bad habits and focus on what my body really needed. Everyone can, step by step, improve their life: this work is my first contribution of what I learned and what I put into practice, all written in a friendly and motivating way to let the reader take action. The choices we make in terms of food and beverages directly affect our microbiome, which is linked to our body and brain. It is a virtuous circle. One you launch your personal project of improvement, you cannot stop it, and you will see a whole different world and live a far better life!

References

Adães, S. (2019, July 8). How The Gut Microbiota Influences Our Immune System. Neurohacker Collective. https://neuro-hacker.com/how-the-gut-microbiota-influences-our-immune-system

Carey, E., & Sarachik, J. (2019, March 7). 10 Processed Foods to Avoid. Healthline; Healthline Media. https://www.health-line.com/health/food-nutrition/processed-foods-to-avoid

Clear, J. (n.d.). The Beginner's Guide to Intermittent Fasting. James Clear. Retrieved August 13, 2020, from https://jamesclear.com/the-beginners-guide-to-intermittent-fast-ing

Corey. (2013, May 9). Frozen Yogurt Covered Blueberries. Family Fresh Meals. https://www.familyfreshmeals.com/2013/05/fro-zen-yogurt-covered-blueberries.html

CROHN'S & COLITIS FOUNDATION. (n.d.). A Look Back at Our Beginning | Crohn's & Colitis Foundation. Crohn's & Colitis Foundation. Retrieved August 13, 2020, from https://www.crohnscolitisfoundation.org/about/our-beginning

Dix, M. (2020, March 26). What's an Unhealthy Gut? How Gut Health Affects You. Healthline; Healthline Media. https://www.healthline.com/health/gut-health

Edermaniger, L. (2019, December 31). How To Improve Gut Health: 16 Simple Hacks For Your Gut In 2020. Atlas Biomed Blog | Take Control of Your Health with No-Nonsense News on Life-style, Gut Microbes and Genetics. https://atlasbio-med.com/blog/16-easy-hacks-to-enhance-your-gut-health-every-day-in-2020/

Edermaniger, L. (2020, February 20). 12 Superfoods For Your Microbiome To Boost Gut Health And Digestion. Atlas Biomed Blog | Take Control of Your Health with No-Nonsense News on

Lifestyle, Gut Microbes and Genetics. https://atlasbio-med.com/blog/superfoods-for-microbiome-health/

Foster, K. (2016, August 8). Recipe: Caprese Avocado Toast. Kitchn. https://www.thekitchn.com/recipe-caprese-avocado-toast-232930

Frothingham, S. (2019, October 24). How Long Does It Take for a New Behavior to Become Automatic? Healthline; Healthline Media. https://www.healthline.com/health/how-long-does-it-take-to-form-a-habit

Gunnars, K. (2018, June 28). 11 Proven Health Benefits of Quinoa. Healthline; Healthline Media. https://www.healthline.com/nutrition/11-proven-benefits-of-quinoa

Gunnars, K. (2018a, July 16). A Low-Carb Meal Plan and Menu to Improve Your Health. Healthline; Healthline Media. https://www.healthline.com/nutrition/low-carb-diet-meal-plan-and-menu

Gunnars, K. (2018b, July 24). Mediterranean Diet 101: A Meal Plan and Beginner's Guide. Healthline. https://www.healthline.com/nutrition/mediterranean-diet-meal-plan

Gunnars, K. (2018c, August 1). The Paleo Diet — A Beginner's Guide + Meal Plan. Healthline. https://www.healthline.com/nutrition/paleo-diet-meal-plan-and-menu

Gunnars, K. (2020, February 12). Top 10 Evidence-Based Health Benefits of Coconut Oil. Healthline. https://www.healthline.com/nutrition/top-10-evidence-based-health-benefits-of-coconut-oil

Heidi. (n.d.-a). Citrus Pan-Seared Shrimp Recipe (Easy Shrimp Dish!) | foodiecrush.com. Foodiecrush. Retrieved August 13, 2020, from https://www.foodiecrush.com/pan-seared-citrus-shrimp-recipe/

Heidi. (n.d.-b). Citrus Shrimp Salad with Avocado | foodiecrush.com. Foodiecrush. Retrieved August 13, 2020, from https://www.foodiecrush.com/citrus-shrimp-avocado-salad/

Jennings, K.-A. (2018, December 17). 10 Impressive Health Benefits of Apples. Healthline; Healthline Media. https://www.healthline.com/nutrition/10-health-benefits-of-apples

Leech, J. (2018, September 14). 11 Proven Benefits of Olive Oil. Healthline. https://www.healthline.com/nutrition/11-proven-benefits-of-olive-oil

Leech, J. (2019, June 11). 11 Evidence-Based Health Benefits of Eating Fish. Healthline. https://www.healthline.com/nutrition/11-health-benefits-of-fish

Lewis, S. (2017, June 3). Probiotics and Prebiotics: What's the Difference? Healthline. https://www.healthline.com/nutrition/probiotics-and-prebiotics

Link, R. (2019, April 4). A Complete Vegan Meal Plan and Sample Menu. Healthline. https://www.healthline.com/nutrition/vegan-meal-plan

Maroney, L. (2019, August 28). Greek Inspired Spinach and Feta Breakfast Wrap. The Spruce Eats. https://www.thespruceeats.com/spinach-and-feta-breakfast-wrap-428353

McDowell, E. (n.d.-a). Cauliflower Rice. PureWow. Retrieved August 13, 2020, from https://www.purewow.com/recipes/Cauliflower-Rice

McDowell, E. (n.d.-b). Whole30 Chicken Meatballs and Cauliflower Rice with Coconut-Herb Sauce. PureWow. Retrieved August 13, 2020, from https://www.purewow.com/recipes/whole30-chicken-meatballs-cauliflower-rice-coconut-herb-sauce

Meixner, M. (2019, May 28). 7 Health Benefits of Grass-Fed Butter. Healthline. https://www.healthline.com/nutrition/grass-fed-butter

Microbiome, T. D. (2019, December 9). 10 Microbiome-Healing Herbs and Spices to Add to Your Meals. Dr. Mahmoud Ghannoum, Ph.D., MBA, FIDSA. https://drmicrobiome.com/gut-friendly/10-microbiome-healing-herbs-and-spices-to-add-to-your-meals/

Microbiome, T. D. (2020, February 12). Gut Reset Diet: How To Restore Gut Health | Dr. Microbiome. Dr. Mahmoud Ghannoum, Ph.D., MBA, FIDSA. https://drmicrobiome.com/health/gut-reset-diet/

NDTV Food, & Borah, P. (2018, August 20). 7 Wonderful Benefits Of Banana: How To Include The Fruit In Your Daily Diet. NDTV Food. https://food.ndtv.com/food-drinks/benefits-of-banana-how-to-include-the-fruit-in-your-daily-diet-1216006

NDTV Food. (2018, June 19). 6 Incredible Benefits of Sunflower Oil. NDTV Food. https://food.ndtv.com/food-drinks/6-incredible-benefits-of-sunflower-oil-1636359

Nutrition Tips for Inflammatory Bowel Disease. (n.d.). Ucsfhealth.Org. Retrieved August 13, 2020, from https://www.ucsfhealth.org/education/nutrition-tips-for-inflammatory-bowel-disease

Osipov, O. (2019, November 4). No Bake Peanut Butter Pie. IFOODreal. https://ifoodreal.com/clean-no-bake-peanut-butter-pie/

Palsdottir, H. (2018, August 28). 11 Probiotic Foods That Are Super Healthy. Healthline. https://www.healthline.com/nutrition/11-super-healthy-probiotic-foods

Petre, A. (2019, January 22). The Microbiome Diet Review: Food Lists, Benefits, and Meal Plan. Healthline. https://www.healthline.com/nutrition/microbiome-diet

Prof Tim Spector. (2020, February 10). 15 tips to boost your gut microbiome. BBC Science Focus Magazine; BBC Science Focus Magazine. https://www.sciencefocus.com/the-human-body/how-to-boost-your-microbiome/

Robertson, PhD, R. (2017, December 1). The 9 Healthiest Beans and Legumes You Can Eat. Healthline. https://www.healthline.com/nutrition/healthiest-beans-legumes

Robertson, R. (2017, June 27). Why the Gut Microbiome Is Crucial for Your Health. Healthline. https://www.healthline.com/nutrition/gut-microbiome-and-health

Running to the Kitchen. (2014, May 30). How to Ferment Vegetables - Make Your Own Fermented Vegetables. Running to the Kitchen®. https://www.runningtothekitchen.com/how-to-ferment-vegetables/

Savin, Z., Kivity, S., Yonath, H., & Yehuda, S. (2018). Smoking and the intestinal microbiome. Archives of Microbiology, 200(5), 677–684. https://doi.org/10.1007/s00203-018-1506-2

SciShow. (2017a). Meet Your Microbiome! [YouTube Video]. In YouTube.
https://www.youtube.com/watch?v=Ybk7E7SLbWw&list=WL&index=11&t=44s

SciShow. (2017b). Your Microbiome and Your Brain [YouTube Video]. In YouTube.
https://www.youtube.com/watch?v=2ycHwcV9MvM&list=WL&index=12&t=0s

Semeco, A. (2016, June 8). The 19 Best Prebiotic Foods You Should Eat. Healthline; Healthline Media. https://www.healthline.com/nutrition/19-best-prebiotic-foods

Sengupta, S. (2018, June 29). Apple Fruit Benefits: 8 Incredible Health Benefits Of Apple That You May Not Have Known. NDTV Food. https://food.ndtv.com/food-drinks/apple-fruit-benefits-8-incredible-health-benefits-of-apple-that-you-may-not-have-known-1761603

Sifferlin, A. (2018, April 12). 10 Foods Filled With Probiotics. Time. https://time.com/5236659/best-probiotic-foods/

Spritzler, F. (2019, April 24). 11 Reasons Why Berries Are Among the Healthiest Foods on Earth. Healthline. https://www.healthline.com/nutrition/11-reasons-to-eat-berries

Wikipedia Contributors. (2019, September 24). Food pyramid (nutrition). Wikipedia; Wikimedia Foundation. https://en.wikipedia.org/wiki/Food_pyramid_(nutrition)